NATURE CURE

Philosophy & Practice Based on the
Unity of Disease & Cure

NATURE CURE
Philosophy & Practice Based on the Unity of Disease & Cure

HENRY LINDLAHR, M.D.

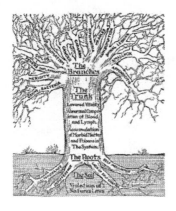

WILDSIDE PRESS

NATURE CURE

A new edition based on the
TWENTIETH EDITION
(1922)

Published by:
Wildside Press
P.O. Box 301
Holicong, PA 18928-0301
www.wildsidepress.com

CONTENTS

"Ho, ye who suffer! Know ye suffer from vowselves. None else compels—no other holds ye that ye live or die."
—*Siddartha*

TO THE PROGRESSIVE
PHYSICIANS OF THE AGE

There are two principal methods of treating disease. One is the combative, the other the preventive. The trend of modern medical research and practice in our great colleges and endowed research institutes is almost entirely along combative lines, while the individual, progressive physician learns to work more and more along preventive lines. The slogan of modern medical science is, "Kill the germ and cure the disease." The usual procedure is to wait until acute or chronic diseases have fully developed, and then, if possible, to subdue them by means of drugs, surgical operations, and by means of the morbid products of disease, in the form of serums, antitoxins, vaccines, etc. The combative method fights disease with disease, poison with poison, and germs with germs and germ products. In the language of the Good Book, it is "Beelzebub against the Devil."

The preventive method does not wait until diseases have fully developed and gained the ascendancy in the body, but concentrates its best endeavors on preventing, by hygienic living and by natural methods of treatment, the development of diseases. By these it endeavors to put the human body in such a normal, healthy condition that it is practically proof against infection or contagion by disease taints and miasms, and against the inroads of germs, bacteria and parasites.

The question is, which method is the most practical, the most successful and most popular? Which will stand the test of "the survival of the fittest" in the great struggle for existence?

The medical profession has good reason to be alarmed by the inroads made in its work by irregular, unorthodox systems, schools and cults of treating human ailments; but instead of raging at the audacious presumption of these interlopers, would it not be better to inquire if there is not some reason for the astonishing spread and popularity of these therapeutic innovations?

Their success undoubtedly is based on the fact that they concentrate their best efforts on preventive instead of combative methods of treating disease. People are beginning to realize that it is cheaper and more advantageous to prevent disease than to cure it. To create and maintain continuous, buoyant good health means greater efficiency for mental and physical work; greater capacity for the true enjoyment of life, and the best insurance against failure and poverty. Therefore, he who builds health is of greater value to humanity than he who allows people to drift into disease through ignorance of Nature's laws, and then attempts to cure them by doubtful and uncertain combative methods.

It is said that in China the physician is hired and paid by the year; that he receives a certain stipend as long as the members of the family are in good health, but that the salary is suspended as long as one of his charges is ill. If some similar method of engaging and paying for medical services were in vogue in this country the trend of medical research and practice would soon undergo a radical change.

The diet expert, the hydropath, the physical culturist, the adjuster of the spine, the mental healer, and Christian scientist, do not pay much attention to the pathological conditions or to the symptoms of disease. They regulate the diet and habits of living on a natural basis, promote elimination, teach correct breathing and wholesome exercise, correct the mechanical lesions of the spine, establish the right mental and emotional attitude and, in so far as they succeed in doing this, they build health and diminish the possibility of disease. The successful doctor of the future will have to fall in line with the procession and do more teaching than prescribing.

I realize that many of the statements and claims made in this volume will seem radical and irrational to my colleagues of the regular school of medicine. They win say that most of my teachings are contrary to the firmly established theories of medical science. All I ask, of them is not to judge too hastily; to observe, to think and to test, and I am certain that they will find verified in actual experience many of the teachings of the Nature Cure Philosophy. Medical science has had to abandon innumerable theories and practices which at one time were as firmly established as some of the pet theories of today.

By none of the statements made in this book do I mean to deny the necessity of combative methods under certain circumstances. What I wish to emphasize is that the regular school of medicine is spending too much of its effort along combative lines and not enough along preventive. It would be foolish to deny the necessity of surgery in traumatism, and in abnormal conditions which require mechanical means of adjustment or treatment.

Such necessity, for instance, will exist in certain obstetrical cases, as long as women have not learned, or are not willing to live in such a way as to make surgical intervention unnecessary in childbirth. The same is true with regard to the treatment of germ diseases. As long as people persist in violating the laws of their being, and thereby making their bodies prolific breeding grounds for disease taints, germs and parasites which are bound to provoke inflammatory, feverish processes (Nature's cleansing and healing efforts), combative measures will have to be resorted to by the physician, and precautionary measures against infection will have to be observed, but these should be in harmony with Nature's endeavors, not contrary and suppressive; they should tend to conserve and not to destroy.

Natural dietetics, fasting, hydropathy, osteopathy, chiropractic, and mental therapeutics, are combative as well as preventive, but if properly applied they do not in any way injure the organism or interfere with Nature's intent and Nature's methods. This cannot be said for much of the surgical and medical treatment of the old school of medicine. We criticize and condemn only those methods which are suppressive and destructive instead of curative.

In many instances already the warnings and teachings of Nature Cure Philosophy have been verified, and had to be heeded and accepted by medical science. The exponents of Nature Cure protested against the barbarous practice of withholding water from patients burning in fever heat, and against the exclusion of fresh air from the sickroom by order of the doctor. The cold water and no drug treatment of typhoid fever, the water treatment for other acute diseases, as well as the open air treatment for tuberculosis, were forced upon the medical profession by the Nature Cure people. For more than half a century the latter have been curing all inflammaory, feverish diseases, from simple colds to scarlet fever, diphtheria, cerebro-spinal meningitis, smallpox, appendicitis, etc., etc., by hydropathy, fasting, and other natural methods, without resorting at all to the use of poisonous drugs, antitoxins and surgical operations.

For many years before the terrible after-effects of X-Ray treatment, of extirpation of the ovaries, the womb, and of other vital organs, became so patent that the physicians of the regular school could not ignore them any longer, Nature Cure physicians had strongly warned against these unnatural practices, and called attention to their destructive after-effects.

As far back as ten years ago, when the X-Rays were in high favor for the treatment of cancer, lupus, and other diseases, I warned against the use of these rays, claiming that their vibratory velocity was too high and powerful, and therefore destructive to the tissues of the human body. Since the failure of the X-Rays and the discovery of Radio-activity, the rays and emanations of radium and other radio-active substances are widely advertised and exploited as therapeutic agents, but these rays also are far beyond the vibratory ranges of the physical body in velocity and power. Therefore, it remains to be seen whether their injurious by and after-effects do not out-weigh in the long run their beneficial effects.

The destructive action of these high power rays, as well as of inorganic minerals, is very slow and insidious, manifesting only in the course of many years. This new field of therapeutics, therefore, has not yet passed the stage of dangerous experimentation.

Inorganic minerals prove injurious and destructive to the tissues of the human body because they are too slow in vibratory velocity, and too coarse in molecular structure.

It is the intent and purpose of this volume to warn against the exploitation of destructive combative methods to the neglect of preventive constructive and conservative methods. If these teachings contribute something toward this end they will fulfil their mission.

The Author
Chicago, Nov., 1913.

INTRODUCTION

It was the following letter from Mr. William Louden to the editor of *"Health Culture"* which prompted the author to issue the *"Nature Cure Magazine"* (published from November, 1907, to October, 1909). In the series of books of which this is the first volume, he will endeavor to collect and systematize all his former writings in the *"Nature Cure Magazine,"* *"Health Culture,"* *"Life and Action,"* the *"Naturopath,"* the *"Volksrath,"* and other publications, and to amplify these by new material obtained through further research and wider experience.

Mr. Albert Turner,
Editor of *"Health Culture."*

DEAR SIR—

I write to ask what you consider the best book or pamphlet to put into the hands of people generally, in regard to the preservation of health. I know ther e are a number of very excellent publications, but as a rule they deal with certain details or phases of the question, and do not begin with the great underlying principles in such a way as to attract and hold the attention of the masses. One advocates one plan, and another an entirely different, and sometimes a directly opposite plan—such as uncooked vs. thoroughly cooked food; a strictly vegetarian diet, and mental culture in place of attention to either, etc. Such a state of affairs makes it confusing to average people and gets them to believe that health reformers are all at sea, and what is good for one is not good for another, or, in common language, "what is one man's meat is another's poison."

Now, I know it is natural, and doubtless best, that there should be a difference of opinion on any question, but at the same time, if any movement is to be crowned with great success, there should be some underlying principles upon which all should agree, and these should be pressed to the forefront, so as to attract and hold the attention of the people, in place of the divergent details upon which they disagree. If these fundamental laws and principles are thoroughly studied and well defined, it may be found that they would explain the discrepancies between the different theories, and that under certain conditions, one plan is best, and that under different conditions another plan is more applicable, etc. The pushing of these fundamental principles to the front would also tend to correct errors into which the different theorists have fallen, and would certainly tend to make the different theories more homogeneous and more easily understood by people in general, than at present.

In my opinion, the general fundamental principles of life and health are what people need to understand more than anything else. Without this, most of the details will be meaningless or at least confusing dogmas. I don't mean by these fundamental principles the details of anatomy, or, for that matter, the details of anything else, but the general rules governing life and death, so that people may know which way they, are tending, and may understand the many illusions with which life and death, as well as all else in nature are beset.

Yours truly,
WILLIAM LOUDEN
Louden Mfg. Co.,
Fairfield, Iowa.

The present volume and others of the "Nature Cure Series" which are to follow are an attempt to answer Mr. Louden's inquiry and to formulate and elucidate the fundamental laws of health, disease and cure for which he and many others have been vainly seeking. Who among you at some time or another, has not thought and felt like Mr. Louden and in doubt and perplexity voiced Pilate's query,

What Is Truth?

The exact information and rational method of teaching which Mr. Louden is seeking, has heretofore been wanting in health-culture literature.

Many, indeed, stand ready and willing to show the way to physical, mental and moral perfection. Hundreds, yes, thousands, of different cults, isms, teachers, books and periodicals treat of these subjects, but their teachings are so manifold, so contradictory and confusing, that one becomes bewildered amid the ever increasing testimony. As is often the case in the study of complicated subjects, the more one reads and the more one hears, the less one knows. I believe that no one has described more strikingly this state of general perplexity than Mr. Louden in his excellent letter.

Nevertheless, these simple fundamental laws and principles really exist. They must exist, because everything in Nature, including the processes of health, of disease and cure, of birth, of life and death, are subject to law and order.

Allopathy, or Old School Medical Science, admits that it does not know these fundamental principles; that it reasons, not from underlying causes, but from external symptoms and personal experiences. It is, therefore, self-confessedly full of doubts, errors and confusion; in short, empirical—and necessarily, a failure.

Many teachers of Nature Cure, Hygiene and Health cults have stumbled accidentally upon some of the natural laws and true methods of healing, but have failed to grasp and to formulate the broad underlying principles. For this reason they are often partly right and partly wrong and very apt to overdo certain methods to the neglect of others just as effective and essential, or even more so.

I shall endeavor in these volumes to formulate and elucidate some of the fundamental laws and principles underlying the phenomena of life and death, health, disease and cure, and shall try to ascertain in the light of these laws how much of truth and how much of error, how much of usefulness and how much of harmfulness there may be contained in the various theories and systems of living and of healing.

Nature Owe an Exact Science

One of the reasons why Nature Cure is not more popular with the medical profession and the public is that it is **too simple.** The average mind is more impressed by the involved and mysterious than by the simple and common-sense.

However, it remains a fact that "exact science" reduces complexity and confusion to simplicity and clearness. Science becomes exact science only when the underlying laws which correlate and unify its scattered facts and theories have been discovered.

These simple laws rightly understood and applied will do for medical science what the law of gravitation has done for physics and astronomy, and what the laws of chemical affinity have done for chemistry, they will place medical science in the ranks of exact sciences. The understanding and proper application of these truths will explain every fact and phenomenon in the processes of health, disease and cure, and will enable the student to reason from simple, natural laws and principles to their logical effects. The "Regular" school of medicine, so far, has endeavored to build a medical science on the observation of "effects" and " experiences," but since one fundamental law of nature may produce a million seemingly differing effects it becomes self-evident that it is utterly impossible to found an exact science on such uncertain and conflicting evidence.

The primary laws and principles once understood, it becomes easy to reason from and to explain through them, the various phenomena which they produce. Herein lie the merit and achievement of the Nature Cure philosophy.

Chapter I

What Is Nature Cure?

It is vastly more than a system of curing aches and pains; **it is a complete revolution in the art and science of living.** It is the practical realization and application of all that is good in natural science, philosophy and religion. Like many another world-wide revolution and reformation, it had its inception in Germany, the land of thinkers and philosophers.

About seventy years ago this greatest and most beneficent of reformation movements was inaugurated by Priessnitz in Grafenberg, a small village in the Silesian mountains. The originator of Nature Cure was a simple farmer, but he had a natural genius for the art of healing.

His pharmacopeia consisted not in poisonous pills and potions but in plenty of exercise, fresh mountain air, water treatments in the cool, sparkling brooks, and simple, wholesome country fare, consisting largely of black bread, vegetables, and milk fresh from cows fed on nutritious mountain grasses.

The results accomplished by these simple means were wonderful. Before he died, a large sanitarium, filled with patients from all over the world and from all stations of life, had grown up around his forest home.

Among those who made the pilgrimage to Grafenberg to become patients and students of this genial healer, the simple-minded farmer-physician, were wealthy merchants, princes and doctors from all parts of the world.

Rapidly the idea of drugless healing spread over Germany and over the civilized world. In the Fatherland, Hahn the apothecary, Kuhne the weaver, Rikli the manufacturer, Father Kneipp the priest, Lahmann the doctor, and Turnvater Jahn, the founder of physical culture, became enthusiastic pupils and followers of Priessnitz.

Each one of these men enlarged and enriched some special field of the great realm of natural healing. Some elaborated the water cure and natural dietetics, others invented various systems of manipulative treatment, earth, air and light cures, magnetic healing, mental therapeutics, curative gymnastics, etc., etc. Von Peckzely added the Diagnosis from the Eye, which reveals not only the innermost secrets of the human organism, but also Nature's ways and means of cure, and the changes for better or for worse continually occurring in the body.

In this country, Dr. Trall of New York, Dr. Jackson of Danville, Dr. Kellogg of Battle Creek, and others caught the infection and crossed the ocean to become students of Priessnitz. The achievements of these men in their respective fields of endeavor will stand as enduring monuments to the eternal truths revealed by the genius of Nature Cure.

Quimby, the itinerant spiritualist and healer, became successful and renowned by the application of the natural methods of cure. At first his favorite methods were water, massage, magnetic and mental treatment. Gradually he concentrated his efforts on metaphysical methods of cure, and before he died, he evolved a complete system of magnetic and mental therapeutics.

Quimby's teachings and methods were adopted by Mrs. Eddy, his most enthusiastic pupil, and by her elaborated into Christian Science, the latest and most successful of modern mental-healing cults.

Dr. Still of Kirksville, Missouri, made a valuable addition to natural methods of treatment by the invention of Osteopathy, a system of scientific manipulation of the bony structures, nerves and nerve centers, muscles and ligaments. A later development of manipulative science is Chiropractic, originated by Dr. Palmer of Davenport, Iowa. Thus the simple pioneers of German Nature Cure, every one of them gifted by Nature with the instinct and genius of the true healer, who is born, not made, laid the foundation for the worldwide modern healthculture movement.

They were not blinded or confused by the conflicting theories of books and authorities, or by the action of a thousand different drugs on a legion of different symptoms, but **applied common-sense reasoning to the solution of the problems of health, disease and cure.**

They went for inspiration to field and forest rather than to the murky atmosphere of the dissecting and vivisection rooms. They studied the whole and not only the parts, **causes as well as effects and symptoms.** Realizing that man had lost his natural instinct and strayed far from Nature's ways, they studied and imitated the natural habits of the animal creation rather than the confusing doctrines of the schools.

Thus they proclaimed the "return to Nature" and the "new gospel of health," which are destined to free humanity from the destructive influences of alcoholism, red meat overeating, the dope and tobacco habit, and of drug poisoning, vaccination, surgical mutilation, vivisection and a thousand other abuses practiced in the name of science.

When parents learn how to create children in accord with natural law, how to mold their bodies and their characters into harmony and beauty **before** the new life sees the light of day, when they learn to rear their offspring in health of body and purity of mind, in harmony with the laws of their being, then we shall have true types of beautiful manhood and womanhood, then children will no longer be a curse and a burden to themselves and to those who bring them into the world or to society at large.

These thoughts are not the mere dreams of a visionary. When we see the wonderful changes wrought in a human being by a few months or years of rational living and treatment, it seems not impossible or improbable that these ideals may be realized within a few generations.

Children thus born and reared in harmony with the law will be the future masters of the earth. They will need neither gold nor influence to win in the race of life—their innate powers of body and soul will make them victors over every circumstance. The offspring of alcoholism, drug poisoning and sexual perversity will cut but sorry figures in comparison with the manhood and womanhood of a true and noble aristocracy of health.

Chapter II

Catechism of Nature Cure

The philosophy of Nature Cure is based on sciences dealing with newly discovered or rediscovered natural laws and principles, and with their application to the phenomena of life and death, health, disease and cure.

Every new science embodying new modes of thought requires exact modes of expression and new definitions of already well-known words and phrases.

Therefore, we have endeavored to define, as precisely as possible, certain words and phrases which convey meanings and ideas peculiar to the teachings of Nature Cure.

The student of Nature Cure and kindred subjects will do well to study these definitions and formulated principles closely, as they contain the pith and marrow of our philosophy and greatly facilitate its understanding.

(1) What Is Nature Cure?

Nature Cure is a system of building the entire being in harmony with the constructive principle in Nature on the physical, mental, moral and spiritual planes of being.

(2) What Is the Constructive Principle in Nature?

The constructive principle in Nature is that principle which builds up, improves and repairs, which always makes for the perfect type, whose activity in Nature is designated as evolutionary and constructive and which is opposed to the destructive principle in Nature

(3) What Is the Destructive Principle in Nature?

The destructive principle in Nature is that principle which disintegrates and destroys existing forms and types, and whose activity in Nature is designated as devolutionary and destructive.

(4) What Is Normal or Natural?

That is normal or natural which is in harmonic relation with the life purposes of the individual and the constructive principle in Nature.

(5) What Is Health?

Health is normal and harmonious vibration of the elements and forces composing the human entity on the physical, mental, moral and spiritual planes of being, in conformity with the constructive principle of Nature applied to individual life.

(6) What Is Disease?

Disease is abnormal or inharmonious vibration of the elements and forces composing the human entity on one or more planes of being, in conformity with the destructive principle of Nature applied to individual life.

(7) What Is the Primary Cause of Disease?

The primary cause of disease, barring accidental or surgical injury to the human organism and surroundings hostile to human life, is **violation of Nature's Laws.**

(8) What Is the Effect of Violation of Nature's Laws on the Physical Human Organism?

The effect of violation of Nature's Laws on the physical human organism are:

1. Lowered vitality.

2. Abnormal composition of blood and lymph.

3. Accumulation of waste matter, morbid materials and poisons.

These conditions are identical with disease, because they tend to lower, hinder or inhibit normal function (harmonious vibration) and because they engender and promote destruction of living tissues.

(9) What Is Acute Disease?

What is commonly called acute disease is in reality the result of Nature's efforts to eliminate from the organism waste matter, foreign matter and poisons, and to repair injury to living tissues. In other words, **every so-called acute disease is the result of a cleansing and healing effort of Nature.** The real disease is lowered vitality, abnormal composition of the vital fluids (blood and lymph) and the resulting accumulation of waste materials and poisons.

(10) What Is Chronic Disease?

1. Chronic disease is a condition of the organism in which lowered vibration (lowered vitality), due to the accumulation of waste matter and poisons, with the consequent destruction of vital parts and organs, has progressed to such an extent that

Nature's constructive and healing forces are no longer able to react against the disease conditions by acute corrective efforts (healing crises).

2. Chronic disease is a condition of the organism in which the morbid encumbrances have gained the ascendancy and prevent acute reaction (healing crises) on the part of the constructive forces of Nature.

3. Chronic disease is the inability of the organism to react by acute efforts or healing crises against constitutional disease conditions.

(11) What Is a Healing Crisis?

A healing crisis is an acute reaction, resulting from the ascendancy of Nature's healing forces over disease conditions. Its tendency is toward recovery, and it is, therefore, in conformity with Nature's constructive principle.

(12) Are All Acute Reactions Healing Crises?

No, there are healing crises and disease crises.

(13) What Is a Disease Crisis?

A disease crisis is an acute reaction resulting from the ascendancy of disease conditions over the healing forces of the organism. Its tendency is toward fatal termination, and it is, therefore, in conformity with Nature's destructive principle

(14) What Is Cure?

Cure is the readjustment of the human organism from abnormal to normal conditions and functions.

(15) What Methods of Cure Are in Conformity with the Constructive Principle in Nature?

Those methods which:

1. Establish normal surroundings and natural habits of life in accord with Nature's Laws.

2. Economize vital force.

3. Build up the blood on a natural basis, that is, supply the blood with its natural constituents in right proportions.

4. Promote the elimination of waste matter and poisons without in any way injuring the human body.

5. Arouse the individual in the highest possible degree to the consciousness of personal accountability and the necessity of intelligent personal effort and self-help.

(16) Are Medicines in Conformity with the Constructive Principle in Nature?

Medicines are in conformity with the constructive principle in Nature insofar as they, in themselves, are not injurious and destructive to the human organism and insofar as they act as tissue foods and promote the neutralization and elimination of morbid matter and poisons.

(17) Are Poisonous Drugs and Promiscuous Surgical Operations in Conformity with the Constructive Principle in Nature?

Poisonous drugs and promiscuous operations are **not** usually in conformity with the constructive principle in Nature, because:

1. They suppress acute diseases or reactions (crises), the cleaning and healing efforts of Nature.

2. They are in themselves harmful and destructive to human life.

3. Such treatment fosters the belief that drugs and surgical operations can be substituted for obedience to Nature's Laws and for personal effort and self-help.

(18) Is Metaphysical Healing in Conformity with the Constructive Principle in Nature?

Metaphysical systems of healing are in conformity with the constructive principle in Nature insofar as:

1. They do not interfere with or suppress Nature's healing efforts.

2. They awaken hope and confidence (therapeutic faith) and increase the inflow of vital force into the organism.

They are **not** in conformity with the constructive principle in Nature in so far as:

1. They fail to assist Nature's healing efforts.

2. They ignore, obscure and deny the laws of Nature and defy the dictates of reason and common sense.

3. They substitute, in the treatment of disease, a blind, dogmatic belief in the wonder-working power of metaphysical formulas and prayer for intelligent cooperation with Nature's constructive forces for personal effort and self-help.

4. They weaken the consciousness of personal responsibility.

(19) Is Nature Cure in Conformity with the Constructive Principle in Nature?

Nature Cure is in conformity with the constructive principle in Nature because:

1. It teaches that the primary cause of weakness and disease is disobedience to the laws of Nature.

2. It arouses the individual to the study of natural laws and demonstrates the necessity of strict compliance with these laws.

3. It strengthens the consciousness of personal responsibility of the individual for his own status of health and for the hereditary conditions, traits and tendencies of his offspring.

4. It encourages personal effort and self-help.

5. It adapts surroundings and habits of life to natural laws.

6. It assists Nature's cleansing and healing efforts by simple natural means and methods of treatment which are in no wise harmful or destructive to health and life, and which are within the reach of everyone.

(20) What Are the Natural Methods of Living and of Treatment?

1. **Return to Nature** by the regulation of eating, drinking, breathing, bathing, dressing, working, resting, thinking, the moral life, sexual and social activities, etc., on a normal and natural basis.

2. **Elementary remedies,** such as water, air, light, earth cures, magnetism, electricity, etc.

3. **Chemical remedies,** such as scientific food selection and combination, specific nutritional augmentation with natural food concentrates, homeopathic medicines, simple herb extracts and the vitochemical remedies.

4. **Mechanical remedies,** such as corrective gymnastics, massage, magnetic treatment, chiropractic or osteopathic manipulation and, when indicated, surgery.

5. **Mental and spiritual remedies,** such as scientific relaxation, normal suggestion, constructive thought, the prayer of faith, etc.

Chapter III

What Is Life?

In our study of the cause and character of disease we must endeavor to begin at the beginning, and that is with LIFE itself, for the processes of health, disease and cure are manifestations of that which we call life, vitality, life elements, etc.

While endeavoring to fathom the mystery of life we soon realize, however, that we are dealing with an ultimate which no human mind is capable of solving or explaining. We can study and understand life only in its manifestations, not in its origin and real essence.

There are two prevalent, but widely differing, conceptions of the nature of life or vital force: the **material** and the **vital.**

The former looks upon life or vital force with all its physical, mental and psychical phenomena as manifestations of the electric, magnetic and chemical activities of the physical-material elements composing the human organism. From this viewpoint, life is a sort of spontaneous combustion, or, as one scientist expressed it, a succession of fermentations.

This materialistic conception of life, however, has already become obsolete among the more advanced biologists as a result of the wonderful discoveries of modern science, which are fast bridging the chasm between the material and the spiritual realms of being.

But medical science, as taught in the regular schools, is still dominated by the old, crude, mechanical conception of vital force and this, as we shall see, accounts for some of its gravest errors of theory and of practice.

The **vital** conception of life, on the other hand, regards it as the primary force of all forces, coming from the great central source of all power.

This force, which permeates, heats and animates the entire created universe, is the expression of the divine will, the "logos," the "word" of the great creative intelligence. It is this divine energy which sets in motion the whirls in the ether, the electric corpuscles and ions that make up the different atoms and elements of matter.

These corpuscles and ions are positive and negative forms of electricity. Electricity is a form of energy. It is **intelligent** energy; otherwise it could not move with that same wonderful precision in the electrons of the atoms as in the suns and planets of the sidereal universe.

This intelligent energy can have but one source: the will and the intelligence of the Creator; as Swedenborg expresses it, "the great central sun of the universe."

If this supreme intelligence should withdraw its energy, the electrical charges (forms of energy) and with it the atoms, elements, and the entire material universe would disappear in the flash of a moment.

From this it appears that crude matter, instead of being the source of life and of all its complicated mental and spiritual phenomena (which assumption, on the face of it, is absurd), is only an expression of the Life Force, itself a manifestation of the great creative intelligence which some call God, others Nature, the Oversoul, Brahma, Prana, etc., each one according to his best understanding.

It is this supreme power and intelligence, acting in and through every atom, molecule and cell in the human body, which is **the true healer,** the vis medicatrix naturæ, which always endeavors to repair, to heal and to restore the perfect type. All that the physician can do is to remove obstructions and to establish normal conditions within and around the patient, so that the healer within can do his work to the best advantage.

Here the Christian Scientist will say: "That is exactly what we claim. All is God, all is mind! There is no matter! **Our** attitude toward disease is based on these facts."

Well, what of it, Brother Scientist? Suppose, in the final analysis, matter is nothing but vibration, an expression of Divine Mind and Will. That, for all practical purposes, does not justify me to deny and to ignore its reality. Because I have an "all-mind" body, is it advisable for me to place myself in the way of an "all-mind" locomotive moving at the rate of sixty miles an hour?

The question is not **what matter is** in the final analysis, but **how matter affects us**. We have to take it and treat it as we find it. We must be as obedient to the laws of matter as to those of the higher planes of being.

Life Is Vibratory

In the final analysis, all things in Nature, from a fleeti g thought or emotion to the hardest piece of diamond or platinum, are modes of motion or vibration. A few years ago physical science assumed that an atom was the smallest imaginable part of a given element of matter;

that although infinitesimally small, it still represented solid matter. Now, in the light of better evidence, we have good reason to believe that there is no such thing as solid matter: that every atom is made up of charges of negative and positive electricity acting in and upon an omnipresent ether; that the difference between an atom of iron and of hydrogen or any other element consists solely in the number of electrical charges or corpuscles it contains, and on the velocity with which these vibrate around one another.

Thus the atom, which was thought to be the ultimate particle of solid matter, is found to be a little universe in itself in which corpuscles of electricity rotate or vibrate around one another like the suns and planets in the sidereal universe. This explains what we mean when we say life and matter are vibratory.

As early as 1863 John Newlands discovered that when he arranged the elements of matter in the order of their atomic weight, they displayed the same relationship to one another as do the tones in the musical scale. Thus modern chemistry demonstrates the verity of the music of the spheres—another visionary concept of ancient mysticism. The individual atoms in themselves, as well as all the atoms of matter in their relationship to one another, are constructed and arranged in exact correspondence with the laws of harmony. Therefore the entire sidereal universe is built on the laws of music.

That which is orderly, lawful, good, beautiful, natural, healthy, vibrates **in unison** with the harmonics of this great "Diapason of Nature"; in other words, it is in alignment with the constructive principle in Nature.

That which is disorderly, abnormal, ugly, unnatural, unhealthy, vibrates **in discord** with Nature's harmonics. It is in alignment with the destructive principle in Nature.

What we call "Inanimate Nature" is beautiful and orderly because it plays in tune with the score of the Symphony of Life. Man alone can play out of tune. This is his privilege, if he so chooses, by virtue of his freedom of choice and action.

We can now better understand the definitions of health and of disease, given in Chapter Two, "Catechism of Nature Cure" as follows:

"Health is normal and harmonious vibration of the elements and forces composing the human entity on the physical, mental, moral and spiritual planes of being, in conformity with the constructive principle of Nature applied to individual life."

"Disease is abnormal or inharmonious vibration of the elements and forces composing the human entity on one or more planes of being, in conformity with the destructive principle of Nature applied to individual life."

The question naturally arising here is, "Normal or abnormal vibration with what?" The answer is that the vibratory conditions of the organism must be in harmony with Nature's established harmonic relations in the physical, mental, moral, spiritual and psychical realms of human life and action.

What Is an Established Harmonic Relation?

Let us see whether we cannot make this clear by a simile. If a watch is in good condition, in harmonious vibration, its movement is so adjusted that it coincides exactly, in point of time, with the rotations of our earth around its axis. The established, regular movement of the earth forms the basis of the established harmonic relationship between the vibrations of a normal, healthy timepiece and the revolutions of our planet. The watch has to vibrate in unison with the harmonics of the planetary universe in order to be normal, or in harmony.

In like manner, everything that is normal, natural, healthy, good, beautiful must vibrate in unison with its correlated harmonics in Nature.

Obedience the Only Salvation

Orthodox medical science attributes disease largely to accidental causes: to chance infection by disease taints, germs or parasites; to drafts, chills, wet feet, etc.

The religiously inclined frequently attribute disease and other tribulations to the arbitrary rulings of an inscrutable Providence.

Christian Scientists tell us that sin, suffering, disease and all other kinds of evil are only errors of mortal mind, or the products of diseased imagination (though this in itself admits the existence of something abnormal or diseased).

Nature Cure philosophy presents a rational concept of evil, its cause and purpose, namely: that it is brought on by violation of Nature's Laws; that it is corrective in its purpose; that it can be overcome only by compliance with the law. There is no suffering, disease or evil of any kind anywhere unless the law has been transgressed somewhere by someone.

These transgressions of the law may be due to ignorance, to indifference or to wilfulness and viciousness. **The effects will always be commensurate with the causes.**

The science of natural living and healing shows clearly that what we call disease is primarily Nature's effort to eliminate morbid matter and to restore the normal functions of the body; that the processes of disease are just as orderly in their way as everything else in Nature; that we must not check or suppress them, but cooperate with them. Thus we learn, slowly and laboriously, the all-important lesson that "obedience to the law" is the only means of prevention of disease, and the only cure.

The Fundamental Law of Cure, the Law of Action and Reaction, and the Law of Crises, as revealed by the Nature Cure philosophy, impress upon us the truth that there is nothing accidental or arbitrary in the processes of health, disease and cure; that every changing condition is either in harmony or in discord with the laws of our being; that only by complete surrender and obedience to the law can we attain and maintain perfect physical health.

Self-Control, the Master's Key

Thus Nature Cure brings home to us constantly and forcibly the inexorable facts of natural law and the necessity of compliance with the law. Herein lies its great educational value to the individual and to the race. The man who has learned to master his habits and his appetites so as to conform to Nature's Laws on the physical plane, and who has thereby regained his bodily health, realizes that personal effort and self-control are the Master's Key to all further development on the mental and spiritual planes of being as well; that self-mastery and unremitting and unselfish personal effort are the only means of self-completion, of individual and social salvation.

The naturist who has regained health and strength through obedience to the laws of his being, enjoys a measure of self-content, gladness of soul and enthusiasm which cannot be explained by the mere possession of physical health. These highest and purest attainments of the human soul are not the results of mere physical well-being, but of the peace and harmony which come only from obedience to the law. Such is the peace which passeth understanding.

TABLE I
THE UNITY OF DISEASE AND TREATMENT

Barring trauma (injury), advancing age and surroundings un-congenial to human life, all causes of disease may be classified as given below.

Violations of Nature's Laws in thinking, breathing, eating, drinking, dressing, working, resting and in moral, sexual and social conduct result in the following:

Primary and Secondary Causes of Disease

Primary Causes

1. **Lowered vitality** due to overwork, nightwork, excesses, overstimulation, poisonous drugs and ill-advised surgical operations.

2. **Abnormal composition of blood and lymph** due to the improper selection and combination of food, and especially the lack of organic mineral salts and other essential nutritional elements.

3. **Accumulation of waste matter, morbid matter and poisons** due to the first two causes, as well as to faulty diet, overeating, the use of alcoholic and narcotic stimulants, drugs [both street and prescription], vaccines, accidental poisoning and, last but not least, to the suppression of acute diseases (Nature's cleansing and healing efforts) by poisonous drugs and surgical operations.

Secondary Causes

1. Hereditary and constitutional taints of sycosis, scrofula, psora, syphilis; mercurianism, cinchonism, iodism and many other forms of chronic poisoning.

2. Fevers, inflammations, skin eruptions, chronic sinus discharges, ulcers, abscesses, germs, bacteria, parasites, etc.

3. Mechanical subluxations, distortions and displacements of bony structures, muscles and ligaments; weakening and loss of reason, will, and self-control resulting in negative, sensitive and subjective conditions which open the way to nervous prostration, control by other personalities (hypnotic influence, obsession, possession); the different forms of insanity, epilepsy, petit mal, etc.

TABLE II
THE UNITY OF DISEASE AND TREATMENT

In correspondence with the three primary causes of disease, **Nature Cure** recognizes the following:

Natural Methods of Treatment

1. Return to Nature, or the establishment of normal habits and surroundings, which necessitates:

    a. Extension of consciousness by popular general and individual education.

    b. The constant exercise of reason, will and self-control.

    c. A return to natural habits of life in thinking, breathing, eating, dressing, working, resting and in moral, sexual and social conduct.

    d. Correction of mechanical defects and injuries by means of massage, chiropractic or osteopathy, surgery and other mechanical methods of treatment.

2. Economy of Vital Force, which necessitates:

    a. Prevention of waste of vital force by the stoppage of all leaks.

    b. Scientific relaxation, proper rest and sleep.

    c. Proper food selection, magnetic treatment, etc.

    d. The right mental attitude.

3. Elimination, which necessitates:

    a. Scientific selection and combination of food and drink.

    b. Judicious fasting.

    c. Hydrotherapy (water cure).

    d. Light and air baths, friction.

    e. Chiropratic or osteopathy, massage, and other manipulative treatment.

    f. Correct breathing, curative gymnastics.

    g. Such medicinal remedies as will build up the blood on a normal basis and supply the system with the all-important mineral salts in organic form.

Chapter IV

The Unity of Disease and Treatment

here exists a close resemblance between the mechanism and the functions of a watch and of the human body. Their well-being is subject to similar underlying laws and principles. Both a watch and a human body may function abnormally as a result of accidental injury or unfavorable external conditions, such as extreme heat or cold, etc. However, in our present study of the causes of disease we shall not consider accidental injury and hostile environment, but confine ourselves to causes arising within the organism itself.

The watch may cease to vibrate in accord with the harmonics of our planetary universe for several reasons. It may lose time or stand still because (1) the wound spring has spent its force, or (2) its parts are not made up of the right constituents, or (3) foreign matter clogs or corrodes its mechanism.

Similarly, there exist three primary causes of disease and of premature death of the physical body. These are:

1. Lowered vitality.

2. Abnormal composition of blood and lymph.

3. Accumulation of morbid matter and poisons.

In the ultimate, **disease and everything else that we designate as evil are the result of transgressions of natural laws** in thinking, breathing, eating, dressing, working, resting, as well as in moral, sexual and social conduct.

In Tables I and II, I have endeavored to present in concise and comprehensive form the primary and the secondary causes or manifestations of disease and the corresponding natural methods of treatment.

In the following chapters I shall endeavor to show that all the different forms, phases and phenomena of disease arising within the human organism, provided they are not caused by accident or external conditions unfavorable to the existence of human life, can be attributed to one or more of three primary causes (as outlined in Tables I and II). When we succeed in proving that all disease originates from a few simple causes, it will not seem so strange and improbable that all disease can be cured by a few simple, natural methods of living and of treatment. If Nature Cure can accomplish this, it establishes its right to be classed with the exact sciences.

The Three Primary Causes of Disease

We shall now consider the three primary causes of disease one by one.

Lowered Vitality

There is a well-defined limit to the running of a watch. When the wound spring has spent its force, the mechanism stops.

So also the living forms of vegetable, animal and human life seem to be wound by Nature to run a certain length of time, in accordance with the laws governing their growth and development. Even the healthiest of animals living in the most congenial surroundings in the freedom of Nature do not much exceed their allotted span of life, nor do they fall much below it. As a rule, the longer the period between birth and maturity, the longer the life of the animal.

All the different families of mammalia, when living in freedom, live closely up to the life period allotted to them by Nature. Man is the only exception. It is claimed that according to the laws of longevity his average length of life should be considerably over one hundred years, while according to life insurance statistics, the average is at present [1913] thirty-seven years. This shows an immense discrepancy between the possible and the actual longevity of man.

Even this brief span of life means little else than weakness, physical and mental suffering and degeneracy for the majority of mankind. Visiting physicians of the public schools in our large cities report that seventy-five percent of all school children show defective health in some way. Diagnosis from the Eye proves that the remaining twenty-five percent are also more or less affected by hereditary and acquired disease conditions. Christian Science says, "There is no disease." Nature's records in the iris of the eye say there is no perfect health.

These established facts of greatly impaired longevity and universal abnormality of the human race would of themselves indicate that there is something radically wrong somewhere in the life habits of man, and that there is ample reason for the great health-reform movement which was started about the middle of the last century by the pioneers of Nature Cure in Germany, and which has since swept, under many different forms and guises, all portions of the civilized world.

When people in general grow better acquainted with the laws underlying prenatal and postnatal child culture, natural living and the natural treatment of diseases, human beings will approach much more closely the normal in health, strength, beauty and longevity. Then will arise a true aristocracy, not of morbid, venous blue blood, but pulsating with the rich red blood of health.

However, to reach this ideal of perfect physical, mental and moral health, succeeding generations will have to adhere to the natural ways of living and of treating their ailments. It cannot be attained by the present generation. The enthusiasts who claim that they can, by their particular methods, achieve perfect health and live the full term of human life, are destined to disappointment. We are so handicapped by the mistakes of the past that the best which most of us adults can do is to patch up, to attain a reasonable measure of health and to approach somewhat nearer Nature's full allotment of life.

Wild animals living in freedom retain their full vigor unimpaired almost to the end of life. Hunters report that among the great herds of buffalo, elk and deer, the oldest bucks are the rulers and maintain their sovereignty over the younger males of the herd solely by reason of their superior strength and prowess. Premature old age, among human beings, as indicated by the early decay of physical and mental powers, is brought on solely by their violation of Nature's Laws in almost all the ordinary habits of life.

Health Positive—Disease Negative

The freer the inflow of life force into the organism, the greater the vitality, the more there is of strength, of positive resisting and recuperating power.

In the book *Harmonics of Evolution* we are told that at the very foundation of the manifestation of life lies the principle of polarity, which expresses itself in the duality and unity of positive and negative affinity. The swaying to and fro of the positive and the negative, the desire to balance incomplete polarity, constitutes the very ebb and flow of life.

Disease is disturbed polarity. Exaggerated positive or negative conditions, whether physical, mental, moral or spiritual, tend to disease on the respective planes of being. Foods, medicines, suggestion and all the other different methods of therapeutic treatment exert on the individual subjected to them either a positive or a negative influence. It is, therefore, of the greatest importance that the physician and every one who wishes to live and work in harmony with Nature's Laws should understand this all-important question of magnetic polarity.

Lowered vitality means lowered, slower and coarser vibration, and this results in lowered resistance to the accumulation of morbid matter, poisons, disease taints, germs and parasites. This is what we designate ordinarily as the negative condition.

Let us see whether we can explain this more fully by a homely but practical illustration: A great many of my readers have probably seen in operation in the summer amusement parks the "human roulette." This contrivance consists of a large wheel, board-covered, somewhat raised in the center, and sloping towards the circumference. The wheel rotates horizontally, evenly with the floor or ground. The merrymakers pay their nickels for the privilege of throwing themselves flat down on the wheel and attempting to cling to it while it rotates with increasing swiftness. While the wheel moves slowly, it is easy enough to cling to it; but the faster it revolves, the more strongly the centrifugal force tends to throw off the human flies who try to stick to it.

The increasing repelling power of the accelerated motion of the wheel may serve as an illustration of that which we call vigorous vibration, good vitality, natural immunity or recuperative power. This is the positive condition.

The more intense the action of the life force, the more rapid and vigorous are the vibratory activities of the atoms and molecules in the cells, and of the cells in the organs and tissues of the body. The more rapid and vigorous this vibratory activity, the more powerful is the repulsion and expulsion of morbid matter, poisons and germs of disease which try to encumber or destroy the organism.

Health and Disease Resident in the Cell

We must not forget that health or disease, in the final analysis, is resident in the cell. Though a minute, microscopic organism, the cell is an independent living being, which is born, grows, eats, drinks, throws off waste matter, multiplies, ages and dies, just like man, the large cell. If the individual cell is well, man, the complex cell, is well also, and vice versa. From this it is apparent that in all our considerations of the processes of health, disease and cure, we have to deal primarily with the individual cell.

The vibratory activity of the cell may be lowered through the decline of vitality brought about in a natural way by advancing age, or in an artificial way through wrong habits of living, wrong thinking and feeling, overwork, unnatural stimulation and excesses of various kinds.

On the other hand, the inflow of vital force into the cells may be obstructed and their vibratory activity lowered by the accumulation of waste and morbid matter in the tissues, blood vessels and nerve channels of the body. Such clogging will interfere with the inflow of life force and with the free and harmonious vibration of the cells and organs of the body as surely as dust in a watch will interfere with the normal action and vibration of its wheels and balances.

From this it is evident that **negative** conditions may be brought about not only by hyperrefinement of the physical organism, but also by clogging it with waste and morbid matter which interfere with the inflow and distribution of the vital force. It also becomes apparent that in such cases the Nature Cure methods of eliminative treatment, such as pure food diet, hydrotherapy, massage, chiropractic, osteopathy, etc., are valuable means of removing these obstructions and promoting the inflow and free circulation of the positive electric and magnetic life currents

Abnormal Composition of Blood and Lymph

As one of the primary causes of disease, we cited abnormal composition of blood and lymph. The human organism is made up of a certain number of elements in well-defined proportions. Chemistry has discovered, so far, about seventeen of these elements in appreciable quantities and has ascertained their functions in the economy of the body. These seventeen elements must be present in the right proportions in order to insure normal texture, structure and functioning of the component parts and organs of the body.

The cells and organs receive their nourishment from the blood and lymph currents. Therefore, these must contain all the elements needed by the organism in the right proportions, and this, of course, depends upon the character and the combination of the food supply.

Every disease arising in the human organism from **internal** causes is accompanied by a deficiency in blood and tissues of certain important mineral elements [organic salts]. Undoubtedly, the majority of these diseases are caused by an unbalanced diet, or by food and drink poisoning. Wrong food combinations, on the one hand, create an overabundance of waste and morbid matter in the system and, on the other hand, fail to supply the positive mineral elements or organic salts on which depends the elimination of waste and systemic poisons from the body.

The great problem of natural dietetics and of natural medical treatment is, therefore, how to restore and maintain the positivity of the blood and of the organism as a whole through providing in food, drink and medicine an abundant supply of the positive mineral salts in organic form.

Accumulation of Morbid Matter and Poisons

This is the third of the primary causes of disease. We have learned how lowered vitality and the abnormal composition of the vital fluids favor the retention of systemic poisons in the body. If, in addition to this, food and drink contain too much of the waste-producing carbohydrates, hydrocarbons and proteins, and not enough of the eliminating positive mineral salts then waste and morbid materials are bound to accumulate in the system and this results in the clogging of the tissues with acid precipitates and earthy deposits.

Such accumulation of waste and morbid matter in blood and tissues creates the great majority of all diseases arising within the human organism. This will be explained fully in the following chapters which deal with the causation of acute and chronic disease.

More harmful and dangerous, and more difficult to eliminate than the different kinds of systemic poisons, that is, those which have originated within the body, are the drug poisons, especially when they are administered in the inorganic mineral form. Health is dependent upon an abundant supply of life force, upon the unobstructed, normal circulation of the vital fluids and upon perfect oxygenation and combustion. Anything that interferes with these essentials causes disease; anything that promotes them establishes health. Nothing so interferes with the inflow of the life force, with free and normal circulation of blood and lymph and with the oxygenation and combustion of food materials and systemic waste as the accumulation of morbid matter and poisons in the tissues of the body.

This I have endeavored to explain more fully in connection with lowered vitality. Let us now see how disease and health are affected by mental and emotional conditions.

Mental and Emotional Influences

Our mental and emotional conditions exert a most powerful influence upon the inflow and distribution of vital force. The author of *The Great Work*[1] has described most graphically in the chapter on Self-Control how fear, worry, anxiety and all kindred emotions create in the system conditions similar to those of freezing; how these destructive vibrations congeal the tissues, clog the channels of life and paralyze the vital functions. He shows how the emotional conditions of impatience, irritability, anger, etc., have a heating, corroding effect upon the tissues of the body.

In like manner, all other destructive emotional vibrations obstruct the inflow and normal distribution of the life forces in and through the organism, while on the other hand the constructive emotions of faith, hope, cheerfulness, happiness and love exert a relaxing, harmonizing influence upon the tissues, blood vessels and nerve channels of the body, thus opening wide the floodgates of the life forces, and raising the discords of weakness, disease and discontent to the harmonics of buoyant health and happiness.

Let us see just how mind controls matter and how it affects the changing conditions of the physical body. Life manifests through vibration. It acts on the mass by acting through its minutest particles. Changes in the physical body are wrought by vibratory changes in atoms, molecules and cells. Health is satisfied polarity, that is, the balancing of the positive and negative elements in harmonious vibration. Anything that interferes with the free, vigorous and harmonious vibration of the minute parts and particles composing the human organism tends to disturb polarity and natural affinity, thus causing discord or disease.

When we fully realize these facts we shall not stand so much in awe of our physical bodies. In the past we have been thinking of the body as a solid and imponderable mass difficult to control and to change. This conception left us in a condition of utter helplessness and hopelessness in the presence of weakness and disease.

We now think of the body as composed of minute corpuscles rotat-

---

1 *The Great Work: The Constructive Principle of Nature in Individual Life,* by John Emmett Richardson {1853-1935}, Indio-American Book Company, Chicago, IL. 1907.

ing around one another within the atom at relatively immense distances. We know that in similar manner the atoms vibrate in the molecule, the molecules in the cell, the cells in the organ and the organs in the body; the whole capable of being changed by a change in the vibrations of its particles.

Thus the erstwhile solid physical mass appears plastic and fluidic, readily swayed and changed by the vibratory harmonies or discords of thoughts and emotions as well as by foods, medicines and therapeutic treatment.

Under the old conception the mind fell readily under the control of the body and became the abject slave of its physical conditions, swayed by fear and apprehension under every sensation of physical weakness, discomfort or pain. The servants lorded it with a high hand over the master of the house, and the result was chaos. Under the new conception, control is placed where it belongs. It is assumed by the real master of the house, the Soul-Man, and the servants, the physical members of the body, remain obedient to his bidding.

This is the new man, the ideal progeny of a new and higher philosophy. Understanding the structure of the body, the laws of its being and the operation of the life elements within it, the superman retains perfect poise and confidence under the most trying circumstances. Animated by an abounding faith in the supremacy of the healing forces within him and sustained by the power of his sovereign will, he governs his body as perfectly as the artist controls his violin and attunes its vibrations to Nature's harmonies of health and happiness.

Chapter V

The Unity of Acute Diseases

In the last chapter I endeavored to explain the three primary causes of disease, namely: (1) **Lowered Vitality**, (2) **Abnormal Composition of Blood and Lymph**, (3) **Accumulation of Waste, Morbid Matter, and Poisons in the System.**

We shall now consider some of the secondary manifestations resulting from these primary causes. Consulting the table on page 30, we find mentioned as the first one of the secondary causes or manifestations of disease, **"Hereditary and Constitutional Taints."**

On first impression, it might be thought that heredity is a primary cause of disease; but on further consideration it becomes apparent that it is an effect and not a primary cause. If the parents possess good vitality and pure, normal blood and tissues, and if they apply in the prenatal and postnatal treatment of the child the necessary insight and foresight, there cannot be disease heredity. In order to create abnormal hereditary tendencies, the parents, or earlier ancestors, must have ignorantly or wantonly violated Nature's Laws, such violation resulting in lowered vitality and in deterioration of blood and tissues.

The female and male germinal cells unite and form the primitive reproductive cell—the prototype of marriage. The human body with its millions of cells and cell colonies is developed by the multiplication, with gradual differentiation, of the reproductive cell. Its abnormalities of structure, of cell materials and of functional tendencies are reproduced just as surely as its normal constituents. Herein lies the simple explanation of heredity which is proved to be an actual fact, not only by common experience and scientific observation but also in a more definite way by Nature's records in the iris of the eye.

The iris of the newborn child reveals in its diagnostic details not only, in a general way, hereditary taints, lowered resistance, and deterioration of vital fluids, but frequently special weakness and deterioration in those organs which were weak or diseased in the parents. Under the conventional (unnatural) management of the infant, these hereditary tendencies to weakness and disease and their corresponding signs in the iris become more and more pronounced, proceeding through the various stages of incumbrance from acute, infantile diseases through chronic catarrhal conditions to the final destructive stages.

In the face of the well-established facts of disease heredity we have, however, this consolation: If the child be treated in accordance with the teachings of Nature Cure philosophy, the abnormal hereditary encumbrances and tendencies can be overcome and eliminated within a few years. If we place the infant organism under the right conditions of living and of treatment, in harmony with the laws of its being, the Life Principle within will approach ever nearer to the establishment of the perfect type. Hundreds of "Nature Cure" babies all over this country are living proofs of this gladsome message to all those who have assumed or intend to assume the responsibilities of parenthood.

Natural Immunity

Under Division II of "Secondary Causes or Manifestations of Disease" we find mentioned germs, bacteria, parasites, inflammations, fevers, skin eruptions, chronic sinus discharges, ulcers, etc.

Modern medical science is built up upon the germ theory of disease and treatment. Since the microscope has revealed the presence and seemingly entirely pernicious activity of certain microorganisms in connection with certain diseases, **it has been assumed that bacteria are the direct, primary causes of most diseases.** Therefore, the slogan now is: "Kill the bacteria (by poisonous antiseptics, serums and antitoxins) and you will cure the disease."

The Nature Cure philosophy takes a different view of the problem. Germs cannot be the cause of disease, because disease germs are also found in healthy bodies. The real cause must be something else. We claim that it is the waste and morbid matter in the system which afford the microorganisms of disease the opportunity to breed and multiply.

We regard microorganisms as **secondary** manifestations of disease, and maintain that bacteria and parasites live, thrive and multiply **to the danger point** in a weakened and diseased organism only. If it were not so, the human family would be extinct within a few months' time.

The fear instilled by the bacterial theory of disease is frequently more destructive than the microorganisms themselves. We have had under observation and treatment a number of insane patients whose peculiar delusion or monomania was an exaggerated fear of germs, a genuine bacteriophobia.

Keep yourself clean and vigorous from within, and you **cannot** be affected by disease taints and germs from without.

Bacteria are practically omnipresent. We absorb them in food and drink, we inhale them in the air we breathe. Our bodies are literally alive with them. The last stages of the digestive processes depend upon the activity of millions of bacteria in the intestinal tract.

The proper thing to do, therefore, is not to try and kill the germs, but to remove the morbid matter and disease taints in which they live.

Instead of concentrating its energies upon killing the germs, whose presence we cannot escape, Nature Cure endeavors to invigorate the system, to build up blood and lymph on a normal basis and to purify the tissues of their morbid encumbrances in such a way as to establish natural immunity to destructive germ activity. Everything that tends to accomplish this without injuring the system by poisonous drugs or surgical operations is good Nature Cure treatment.

To adopt the germ-killing process without purifying and invigorating the organism would be like trying to keep a house free from fungi and vermin by sprinkling it daily with carbolic acid and other germ killers, instead of keeping it pure and sweet by flooding it with fresh air and sunshine and applying freely and vigorously broom, brush and plenty of soap and water. Instead of purifying it, the antiseptics and germ killers would only add to the filth in the house.

All bacteriologists are unanimous in declaring that the various disease germs are found not only in the bodies of the sick, but also in seemingly healthy persons.

A celebrated French bacteriologist reports that in the mouth of a healthy infant, two months old, he found almost all the disease germs known to medical science. Only lately, a celebrated physician, appointed by the French government to investigate the causes of tuberculosis, declared before a meeting of the International Tuberculosis Congress in Rome that he found the bacilli of tuberculosis in ninety-five percent of all the school children he had examined.

Dr. Osler, one of the greatest living medical authorities, mentions repeatedly in his works that the bacilli of diphtheria, pneumonia and of many other virulent diseases are found in the bodies of healthy persons.

The inability of bacteria, by themselves, to create diseases is further confirmed by the well-known facts of natural immunity to specific infection or contagion. All mankind is more or less affected by hereditary and acquired disease taints, morbid encumbrances and drug poisoning, resulting from age-long violation of Nature's Laws and from the suppression of acute diseases; but even under the almost universal present conditions of lowered vitality, morbid heredity and physical and mental degeneration it is found that under identical conditions of exposure to drafts or infection, a certain percentage of individuals only will take the cold or catch the disease. The fact of natural immunity is constantly confirmed by common experience as well as in the clinics and laboratories of our medical schools and research institutes. Of a specific number of mice or rabbits inoculated with particles of cancer, only a small percentage develops the malignant growth and succumbs to its ravages.

The development of infectious and contagious diseases necessitates a certain predisposition, or, as medical science calls it, "disease diathesis." **This predisposition to infection and contagion consists in the primary causes of disease,** which we have designated as lowered vitality, abnormal composition of blood and lymph, and the accumulation of waste, morbid matter and poisons in the system.

Bacteria: Secondary, Not Primary, Manifestations of Disease

In a previous chapter we learned how lowered vitality weakens the resistance of the system to the attacks and inroads of disease germs and poisons. The growth and multiplication of microorganisms depend furthermore upon a congenial, morbid soil. Just as the ordinary yeast germ multiplies in a sugar solution only, so the various microorganisms of disease thrive and multiply to the danger point only in their own peculiar and congenial kind of morbid matter. Thus, the typhoid fever bacillus thrives in a certain kind of effete matter which accumulates in the intestines; the pneumonia bacilli flourish best in the catarrhal secretions of the lungs, and meningitis bacilli in the diseased meninges of the brain and spinal cord.

Dr. Pettenkofer, a celebrated physician and professor of the University of Vienna, also arrived at the conclusion that bacteria, by themselves, cannot create disease, and for years he defended his opinion from the lecture platform and in his writings against the practically solid phalanx of the medical profession. One day he backed his theory by a practical test. While instructing his class in the bacteriological laboratory of the university, he picked up a glass which contained millions of live cholera germs and swallowed its contents before the eyes of the students. The seemingly dangerous experiment was followed only by a slight nausea. Lately I have heard repeatedly of persons in this country who subjected themselves in similar manner to infection, inoculation and contagion with the most virulent kinds of bacteria and disease taints without developing the corresponding diseases.

A few years ago Dr. Rodermund, a physician in the State of Wisconsin, created a sensation all over this country when he smeared his body with the exudate of smallpox sores in order to demonstrate to his medical colleagues that a healthy body could not be infected with the disease. He was arrested and quarantined in jail, but not before he had come in contact with many people. Neither he nor anyone else exposed by him developed smallpox.

During the ten years that I have been connected with sanitarium work, my workers and myself, in giving the various forms of manipulative treatment, have handled intimately thousands of cases of infectious and contagious diseases, and I do not remember a single instance where any one of us was in the least affected by such contact. Ordinary cleanliness, good vitality, clean blood and tissues, the organs of elimination in good, active condition and, last but not least, a positive, fearless attitude of mind will practically establish natural immunity to the inroads and ravages of bacteria and disease taints. If infection takes place, the organism reacts to it through inflammatory processes, and by means of these endeavors to overcome and eliminate microorganisms and poisons from the system.

In this connection it is of interest to learn that the danger to life from bites and stings of poisonous reptiles and insects has been greatly exaggerated. According to popular opinion, anyone bitten by a rattlesnake, gila monster or tarantula is doomed to die, while as a matter of fact the statistics show that only from two to seven percent succumb to the effects of the wounds inflicted by the bites of poisonous reptiles.

In this, as in many other instances, popular opinion should rather be called "popular superstition."

In the open discussions following my public lectures, I am often asked: "What is the right thing to do in case of snakebite? Would you not give plenty of whiskey to save the victim's life?"

It is my belief that of the seven percent who die after being bitten by rattlesnakes or other poisonous snakes, a goodly proportion give up the ghost because of the effects of the enormous doses of strong whiskey that are poured into them under the mistaken idea that the whiskey is an efficient antidote to the snake poison.

People do not know that the death rate from snakebite is so very low, and therefore they attribute the recoveries to the whiskey, just as recoveries from other diseases under medical or metaphysical treatment are attributed to the virtues of the particular medicine or method of treatment instead of to the real healer, the *vis medicatrix naturæ,* the healing power of Nature, which in ninety-three cases in a hundred eliminates the rattlesnake venom without injury to the organism.

To recapitulate: Just as yeast cells are not only the cause but also the product of sugar fermentation, so disease germs are not only a cause (secondary) but also a product of morbid fermentation in the system. Furthermore, just as yeast germs live on and decompose sugar, so disease germs live on and decompose morbid matter and systemic poisons.

In a way, therefore, microorganisms are just as much the product as the cause of disease and act as scavengers or eliminators of morbid matter. In order to hold in check the destructive activity of bacteria and to prevent their multiplication beyond the danger point, Nature resorts to inflammation and manufactures her own antitoxins.

On the other hand, whatever tends to build up the blood on a natural basis, to promote elimination of morbid matter and thereby to limit the activity of destructive microorganisms without injuring the body or depressing its vital functions, is good Nature Cure practice. The first consideration, therefore, in the treatment of inflammation must be to not interfere with its natural course.

By the various statements and claims made in this chapter, I do not wish to convey the idea that I am opposed to scrupulous cleanliness or surgical asepsis. Far from it! These are dictates of common sense. But I do affirm that the danger from germ and other infectious diseases lies just as much or more so in internal filth as in external uncleanliness. Cleanliness and asepsis must go hand in hand with the purification of the inner man in order to insure natural immunity.

Chapter VI

The Laws of Cure

This brings us to the consideration of acute inflammatory and feverish diseases. From what has been said, it follows that inflammation and fever are not primary, but secondary, manifestations of disease. There cannot arise any form of inflammatory disease in the system unless there is present some enemy to health which Nature is endeavoring to overcome and get rid of. On this fact in Nature is based what I claim to be the fundamental Law of Cure.

"Give me fever and I can cure every disease." Thus Hippocrates the Father of Medicine, expressed the fundamental Law of Cure over two thousand years ago. I have expressed this law in the following sentence: **"Every acute disease is the result of a cleansing and healing effort of Nature."**

This law, when thoroughly understood and applied to the treatment of diseases, will in time do for medical science what the discovery of other natural laws has done for physics, astronomy, chemistry and other exact sciences. It will transform the medical empiricism and confusion of the past and present into an exact science by demonstrating the unity of disease and treatment.

Applying the law in a general way, it means that all acute diseases, from a simple cold to measles, scarlet fever, diphtheria, smallpox, pneumonia, etc., represent Nature's efforts to repair injury or to remove from the system some kind of morbid matter, virus, poison or microorganism dangerous to health and life. In other words, acute diseases cannot develop in a perfectly normal, healthy body living under conditions favorable to human life. The question may be asked: "If acute diseases represent Nature's healing efforts, why is it that people die from them?" The answer to this is: the vitality may be too low, the injury or morbid encumbrance too great or the treatment may be inadequate or harmful, so that Nature loses the fight; still, the acute disease represents an **effort** of Nature to overcome the enemies to health and life and to reestablish normal, healthy conditions.

It is a curious fact that this fundamental principle of Nature Cure and Law of Nature has been acknowledged and verified by medical science. The most advanced works on pathology admit the constructive and beneficial character of inflammation. However, when it comes to the **treatment** of acute diseases, physicians seem to forget entirely this basic principle of pathology, and treat inflammation and fever as though they were, in themselves, inimical and destructive to health and life.

From this inconsistency in theory and practice arise all the errors of allopathic medical treatment. Failure to understand this fundamental Law of Cure accounts for all the confusion on the part of the exponents of the different schools of healing sciences, and for the greater part of human suffering.

The Nature Cure philosophy never loses sight of the fundamental Law of Cure. While allopathy regards acute disease conditions as in themselves harmful and hostile to health and life, as something to be cured (we should say suppressed) by drug or knife, the Nature Cure school regards these forcible housecleanings as beneficial and necessary, so long, at least, as people will continue to disregard Nature's Laws. While, through its simple, natural methods of treatment, Nature Cure easily modifies the course of inflammatory and feverish processes and keeps them within safe limits, it never checks or suppresses these acute reactions by poisonous drugs, serums, antiseptics, surgical operations, suggestion or any other suppressive treatment.

Skin eruptions, boils, ulcers, catarrhs, diarrheas, and all other forms of inflammatory febrile disease conditions are indications that there is something hostile to life and health in the organism which Nature is trying to remove or overcome by these so-called "acute" diseases. What, then, can be gained by suppressing them with poisonous drugs and surgical operations? Such practice does not allow Nature to carry on her work of cleansing and repair and to attain her ends. The morbid matter which she endeavored to eliminate by acute reactions is thrown back into the system. Worse than that, drug poisons are added to disease poisons. Is it any wonder that fatal complications arise, or that the acute condition is changed to chronic disease?

Why Does the Greater Part of Allopathic Materia Medica Consist of Virulent Poisons?

The statements made in the preceding pages are a severe indictment of regular medical science, but they point out the difference in the basic principles of the "Old School" of healing and those of the Nature Cure philosophy.

The fundamental Law of Cure quoted in this chapter explains why allopathic medical science is in error, not in a few things only, but in most things. The foundation, the orthodox conception of disease being wrong, it follows that everything which is built thereon must be wrong also.

No matter how learned a man may be, if he begins a problem in arithmetic with the proposition 2x2=5, he never will arrive at a correct solution if he continue to figure into all eternity. Neither can allopathy solve the problem of disease and cure as long as its fundamental conception of disease is based on error.

The fundamental law of cure explains also why the great majority of allopathic prescriptions contain virulent poisons in some form or another and why surgical operations are in high favor with the disciples of the regular school.

The answer of allopathy to the question, "Why do you give poisons?" usually is, "Our materia medica contains poisons because drug poison kills and eliminates disease poison." We, however, claim that drug poisons merely serve to paralyze vital force, whereby the deceptive results of allopathic treatment are obtained.

The following will explain this more fully. We have learned that so-called acute diseases are Nature's cleansing and healing efforts. All acute reactions represent increased activity of vital force, resulting in feverish and inflammatory conditions, accompanied by pain, redness, swelling, high temperature, rapid pulse, catarrhal discharges, skin eruptions, boils, ulcers, etc.

Allopathy regards these violent activities of vital force as detrimental and harmful in themselves. Anything which will inhibit the action of vital force will, in allopathic parlance, cure (?) acute diseases. As a matter of fact, nothing more effectively paralyzes vital force and impairs the vital organs than poisonous drugs and the surgeon's knife. These, therefore, must necessarily constitute the favorite means of cure (?) of the regular school of medicine.

This school mistakes effect for cause. It fails to see that the local inflammation arising within the organism is not the disease, but merely marks the locality and the method through which Nature is trying her best to discharge the morbid encumbrances; that the acute reaction is local, but that its causes or feeders are always constitutional and must be treated constitutionally. When, under the influence of rational, natural treatment, the poisonous irritants are eliminated from blood and tissues, the local symptoms take care of themselves; it does not matter whether they manifest as pimple or cancer, as a simple cold or as consumption.

The Law of Dual Effect

Everywhere in Nature rules the great Law of Action and Reaction. All life sways back and forth between giving and receiving, between action and reaction. The very breath of life mysteriously comes and goes in rhythmical flow. So also heaves and falls in ebb and tide the bosom of Mother Earth.

In some of its aspects, this law is called the Law of Compensation, or the Law of Dual Effect. On its action depends the preservation of energy.

The Great Master expressed the ethical application of this law when he said:

"Give, and it shall be given unto you. . . . For with the same measure that ye mete it shall be measured to you again."—Luke 6:38.

In the realms of physical nature, giving and receiving, action and reaction balance each other mechanically and automatically. What we gain in power we lose in speed or volume, and vice versa. This makes it possible for the mechanic, the scientist and the astronomer to predict with mathematical precision for ages in advance the results of certain activities in Nature.

The great Law of Dual Effect forms the foundation of the healing sciences. It is related to and governs every phenomenon of health, disease and cure. When I formulated the fundamental Law of Cure in the words, **"Every acute disease is the result of a healing effort of Nature,"** this was but another expression of the great Law of Action and Reaction. What we commonly call crisis, acute reaction or acute disease is in reality Nature's attempt to establish health.

Applied to the physical activity of the body, the Law of Compensation may be expressed as follows: "Every agent affecting the human organism produces two effects: a first, apparent, temporary effect, and a second, lasting effect. The secondary, lasting effect is always contrary to the primary, transient effect."

For instance: The first and temporary effect of cold water applied to the skin consists in sending the blood to the interior; but in order to compensate for the local depletion, Nature responds by sending greater quantities of blood back to the surface, resulting in increased warmth and better surface circulation.

The first effect of a hot bath is to draw the blood to the surface; but the secondary effect sends the blood back to the interior, leaving the surface bloodless and chilled.

Stimulants, as we shall see later on, produce their deceptive effects by burning up the reserve stores of vital energy in the organism. This is inevitably followed by weakness and exhaustion in exact proportion to the previous excitation.

The primary effect of relaxation and sleep is weakness, numbness and death-like stupor; the secondary effect, however, is an increase of vitality.

The Law of Dual Effect governs all drug action. The first, temporary, violent effect of poisonous drugs, when given in physiological doses, is usually due to Nature's efforts to overcome and eliminate these substances. The secondary, lasting effect is due to the retention of the drug poisons in the system and their action on the organism.

In theory and practice, allopathy considers the first effect only and ignores the lasting aftereffects of drugs and surgical operations. It administers remedies whose first effect is **contrary** to the disease condition. Therefore, in accordance with the Law of Action and Reaction, the secondary, lasting effect of such remedies must be **similar** to or like the disease condition.

Common, everyday experience should teach us that this is so, for laxatives and cathartics always tend to produce chronic constipation.

The secondary effect of stimulants and tonics of any kind is increased weakness, and their continued use often results in complete exhaustion and paralysis of mental and physical powers.

Headache powders, pain killers, opiates, sedatives and hypnotics may paralyze brain and nerves into temporary insensibility; but, if due to constitutional causes, the pain, nervousness and insomnia will always return with redoubled force. If taken habitually, these agents invariably tend to create heart disease and paralysis, and ultimately develop the patient into a dope fiend.

Cold and catarrh cures (?), such as quinine, coal-tar products, etc., suppress Nature's efforts to eliminate waste and morbid matter through the mucous linings of the respiratory tract, and drive the disease matter back into the lungs, thus breeding pneumonia, chronic catarrhs, asthma and consumption.

Mercury, iodine and all other alteratives, by suppression of external elimination, create **internal** chronic diseases of the most dreadful types, such as locomotor ataxy, paresis, etc.

So the recital might be continued all through orthodox materia medica. Each drug breeds new disease symptoms which are in their turn cured (?) by other poisons, until the insane asylum or merciful death rings down the curtain on the tragedy of a ruined life.

The teaching and practice of homeopathy, as explained in Chapter Twenty-Six, is fully in harmony with the Law of Action and Reaction. Acting upon the basic principle of homeopathy: *Similia similibus curantur,* or like cures like, it administers remedies whose first, temporary effect is similar to the disease conditions. In accordance with the Law of Dual Effect, then, the secondary effect of these remedies must be **contrary** to the disease conditions, that is, curative.

Chapter VII

Suppression Versus Elimination

My claim **that the conventional treatment of acute diseases is suppressive and not curative** will probably be denied by my medical colleagues. They will maintain that their methods also are calculated to eliminate morbid matter and disease germs from the system.

But what are the facts in actual practice? Is it not true that preparations of mercury, lead, zinc and other powerful poisons are constantly used to suppress skin eruptions, boils, abscesses, etc., instead of allowing Nature to rid the system through these skin diseases of scrofulous, venereal and psoric taints?

Some time ago Dr. Wiley, the former Government Chemist, published the ingredients of a number of popular remedies for colds, coughs and catarrh. Every one of them contained some powerful opiate or astringent. These poisonous drugs relieve the cough and the catarrhal conditions by paralyzing the eliminative activity of the membranous linings of the nasal passages, the bronchi and lungs, the digestive and genitourinary organs; but in doing so, they throw back into the system the morbid matter which Nature is trying to get rid of, and add drug poisons to disease poisons.

Equally harmful is suppression by means of the surgeon's knife. It may be a quicker and apparently more effective process to **remove** the inflamed appendix or the diseased tonsils than to cure them by building up the blood and inducing elimination of systemic poisons by natural methods. But operative treatment is not eliminative. It does not remove from the system the original cause of the inflammation or deterioration of tissues and organs, but it does remove the outlet which Nature had established for the escape of morbid materials.

These morbid encumbrances, forcibly retained in the body, weaken and destroy other parts and organs, or affect the general health of the patient.

My own observations during nearly fifteen years of practical experience, confirmed by many other conscientious observers among Nature Cure practitioners as well as physicians of other schools and of allopathy itself, prove positively that the average length of life after a major operation, performed on important, vital parts and organs, is less than ten years, and that after such an operation the general health of the patient is in the great majority of cases not as good as before.

In the following paragraphs are mentioned some very common instances of suppression and some of their usual chronic aftereffects (sequelae).

- **Diarrhea** is suppressed with laudanum and other opiates, which paralyze the peristaltic action of the bowels and, if repeated, soon produce chronic constipation. Gonorrheal discharges and syphilitic ulcers are checked and suppressed by local injections, cauterization and by prescriptions containing mercury, iodine and other poisonous alternatives which effectually prevent Nature's efforts to eliminate the venereal poisons from the system.
- **Gonorrheal discharges and syphilitic ulcers** are checked and supressed by local injections, cauterizatin, and by prescriptions containing mercury, iodine, and other poisonous alternatives which effectually prevent Nature's efforts to elminate the venereal poisons from the system.
- **All feverish diseases** are more or less interfered with or suppressed by antiseptics, antipyretics, serums and antitoxins. The best books on *Materia Medica* and the professors in the colleges teach that these remedies lower the fever because they are "protoplasmic poisons"; because they paralyze the red and white blood corpuscles, benumb heart action and respiration, and depress all vital functions.
- **Nervousness, sleeplessness and pain** are suppressed by sedatives, opiates and hypnotics. Every one of the drugs used for such purposes is a powerful poison which paralyzes brain and nerve action, in that way interfering with Nature's healing efforts and frequently preventing the consummation of beneficial healing crises.
- **Epileptic attacks** and other forms of convulsions are suppressed, but never cured, by bromides which benumb and paralyze the brain and nerve centers. All that these sedatives accomplish is to produce in the course of time idiocy and the different forms of paralysis and premature senility.

  However, is he not considered the best doctor who can most promptly produce these and many similar deceptive results through artificial inhibition or stimulation by means of the most virulent poisons found on earth?
- **Dandruff and falling hair** are caused by the elimination of systemic poisons through the scalp. The thing to do, therefore, is **not to suppress this elimination** and thereby cause the accu-

mulation of poisons in the brain, **but to stop the manufacture of poison in the body and to promote its removal through the natural channels.**

Dandruff cures and hair tonics contain glycerine, poisonous antiseptics and stimulants which are absorbed by scalp and brain, causing dizziness, headaches, loss of memory, neurasthenia, deafness, weakness of sight, etc.

• **Head lice** and similar parasites peculiar to other parts of the body live on scrofulous and psoriotic taints. When these are consumed, the lice depart as they came, no one knows whence or whither.

This is confirmed by the fact that these noxious pests do not remain with all people who have been exposed to them, but only with those whose internal or external filth conditions furnish the parasites with the means of subsistence.

In a number of instances we have seen "healing crises" take the form of lice. At that time the patients were living in the most clean surroundings, taking different forms of water treatment every day and infection was practically impossible.

These people invariably recalled that they had been infested with parasites at some previous time, and that strong antiseptics, mercurial salves, or other means of suppression had been applied.

We prescribe for the removal of lice only cold water and the comb. Even antiseptic soaps should be avoided.

The Results of Suppression of Children's Diseases

• **Sycotic eruptions** on the heads and bodies of infants, also called milk scurf, if suppressed by salves, cream, unsalted butter or merely by warm bathing, are often followed by chorea (St. Vitus' dance), epilepsy, a scrofulous constitution and in later life by tuberculosis.

• **Measles, scarlet fever, diphtheria, spinal meningitis** and other febrile diseases of childhood, if properly treated by natural methods, are curative or at least corrective in their effects on the system, and represent well-defined, orderly natural processes for the elimination of inherited or acquired disease taints, drug poisons, etc. But if arrested or suppressed before they have run their natural course, before Nature has had time to reestablish normal conditions, then the abnormal condition becomes fixed and permanent (chronic).

In addition to this, the poisons and serums employed to arrest the disease process very often affect vital parts and organs permanently, causing the gradual deterioration of cells and tissues, and paving the way for tuberculosis, chronic affection of the kidneys, cancer, etc., in later years.

These self-evident facts, which can be verified by any unprejudiced observer, account for the "mysterious sequelae" of drug- and serum-treated acute diseases, which never occur where natural methods of healing have been correctly employed. Some of these chronic aftereffects are deafness, blindness, heart and kidney diseases, nervous affections, idiocy, infantile paralysis, etc.

These are merely a few ordinary examples of the results of suppression. They could be multiplied a hundred fold, yet medical science assures us that the causes of cancer and other malignant diseases are unknown.

Good Nature Cure Doctrine from an Allopathic Authority

The following utterances of the late Dr. Nicholas Senin strongly confirm our claims as to the nature and cure of disease. Coming from the lips of a celebrated surgeon and physician, these statements should carry some weight with those who, being unable to reason for themselves, worship at the feet of "authority." The quotations referred to are taken from the report of an interview granted by the doctor to Chicago newspaper representatives on his return from his trip around the world.

[*Chicago American*, August 5th, 1906.]
GERMS PLANTED BY TIGHT LACING
Over-Feeding and Over-Dressing
Given as Causes of Cancer

"Dr. Nicholas Senn brought back from Africa, from whence he returned to Chicago yesterday, confirmations of his belief that cancer is a 'civilized' disease.

"Dr. Senn spent from $2,000 to $3,000 worth of time—at the cash value per hour of his time on his first day at home in four months—telling a half dozen newspaper men more than all the world, except himself and a score of specialists like him, know about the fearful disease. He summed up his own learning in the statement that the disease is still incurable except by the knife in its incipient stages and that the best preventive is clean, plain living.

"His investigations of the natives of Africa served to strengthen his conviction that cancer is a product of civilization, 'like apoplexy and scores of other exotic ailments,' Dr. Senn said. He could not find or hear of a case of cancer among the 'Hamites,' as he termed them. And from the fact that he found the disease, to be an unknown one to the Esquimaux of Greenland, he is assured that climate has nothing whatever to do with it. Climate did not cause it, and climate will not cure it.

Cancer Caused by Over-Living

"'The nearer the human race approaches the animals in habits and particularly in the matter of diet and dress, the freer it is from cancer,' he said. 'Cancer comes from over-feeding and over-living.

"'Drinking, gourmandizing, unnatural habits of women, like lacing, all those things help to plant the seeds of cancer in the child.

"'And as we have not learned to cure it the best thing to do is to prevent it when we can. If children were brought up in simplicity by natural mothers; then, if care should be taken to prevent hypernutrition, there would be much less danger from cancer. Cancer itself is an over-fed thing—tissue that never matures, for if I could mature the cells I could cure the disease. The thing for people to do who fear they may have inherited it, is to live simply—there are many cases among people with a tendency to obesity to one among those of a scanty habit of living—and particularly to remove all sources of irritation, like bad teeth, tobacco, and clothes that chafe.'

Studies African Race

"Besides his hobby, as he calls it, Dr. Senn studied the African generally in his voyage along the East Coast of that continent.

"'It was a fine trip,' he said, 'with so many things to learn. Ethnologically I am certain Africans are of common stock. The negro is a negro wherever you find him. From Kaffir to Bushman and pygmy they are all Hamites.

"'They are mostly a fine people physically, lean and tall, except the dwarfs. There is little tendency toward obesity; they have no apoplexy, no distended veins as we have in civilization. Hence their freedom from cancer. They live naturally, and are vegetarians mostly, while the Northern Esquimaux are meat-eaters, but both races eat naturally to sustain life, hence their immunity from that disease. It is where eating is made an art that cancer is most prevalent.

"'They are free from many other diseases that pester us also. Tuberculosis is hardly known, and only along the coast, where it has been taken by the whites. The real curse of the coast country is malaria. It is bad all up and down the East shore. I kept away from it myself by taking five grains of quinine and the juice of a lemon once a day on an empty stomach. That is a good remedy for malaria, for in all my running around I have never had it.'"

(Editor's Note.—Dr. Senn died January 2, 1908. The papers stated after his death, that the doctor had never been well since the return from his long voyage, that his heart and nervous system had been seriously affected by the altitudes of the Andes and of other mountains. We wonder whether the "high altitudes" or the "five grains of quinine daily" were to blame for the celebrated physician's heart disease and death.)

Suppression, the Cause of Chronic Diseases

Dr. Senn was right. If men and women lived more naturally, the majority of diseases would disappear.

The primary cause of disease is violation of Nature's Laws. "Civilization" has largely stood for artificiality of life and for unnatural habits. A higher civilization, yet to come, will combine the most exquisite culture of heart and mind with true simplicity and naturalness of living. Excessive meat eating, strong spices and condiments, alcohol, coffee, tea, overwork, night work, fear, worry, sensuality, corsets, high heels, foul air, improper breathing, lack of exercise, loveless marriages, race suicide, all of these and many other evils of hypercivlization have contributed their share in creating the universal degeneracy of civilized nations commented upon by Dr. Senn.

When the unnatural habits of life alluded to have lowered the vitality and favored the accumulation of waste matter and poisons to such an extent that the sluggish bowels, kidneys, skin and the other organs of elimination are unable to keep a clean house, Nature has to resort to other, more radical means of purification or we should choke in our own impurities. These forcible housecleanings of Nature are colds, catarrh, skin eruptions, diarrheas, boils, ulcers, abnormal perspiration, hemorrhages and many other forms of inflammatory febrile diseases.

Sulphur and mercury may drive back the skin eruptions,

antipyretics and antiseptics may suppress fever and catarrh. The patient and the doctor may congratulate themselves on a speedy cure; but what is the true state of affairs? Nature has been thwarted in her work of healing and cleansing. She had to give up the fight against disease matter in order to combat the more potent poisons of mercury, quinine, iodine, strychnine, etc. **The disease matter is still in the system, plus the drug poison.**

Proof positive of the retention of drug poisons in the organism is furnished by the **Diagnosis from the Eye.** This will be explained more fully in another chapter.

When vitality has been sufficiently restored, Nature may make another attempt at purification, this time, possibly, in another direction; but again her well-meant efforts are defeated. This process of suppression is repeated over and over again until blood and tissues become so loaded with waste material and poisons that the healing forces of the organism can no longer react against them by acute diseases. Then results the chronic condition, which in the vocabulary of the "Old School" of medicine is only another name for incurable disease.

The more skilled the allopathic school becomes in the suppression and prevention of acute diseases by drugs, knife, X-Rays, serums, vaccination virus, etc., the greater will be the increase of chronic dyspepsia, nervous prostration, insanity, locomotor ataxy, paresis, cancer, secondary and tertiary syphilis, tuberculosis and many other so-called incurable diseases. Thus, the standard medical practice is self-supporting; the treatment of acute conditions assuring a lifelong supply of chronic conditions for the doctor to treat.

Suppression of acute diseases, by drugs and knife, is the all-important factor in the creation of malignant diseases which Dr. Senn had overlooked in his discourse on the causes of distructive ailments. If he had steudied his experiences in foreign lands in the light of these explanations he would have found that these scourges of mankind exist only in those parts of earth where the drug store flourishes.

These statements may seem exaggerated; but allow me to cite a few typical cases of suppression and their effects upon the system from our daily practice.

Paresis, locomotor ataxy and paralysis agitans are not, as is usually assumed, due to secondary and tertiary syphilis, **but to the mercury administered for the cure of luetic and other diseases.** In less than six months' time we cure the so-called specific diseases by our natural methods, provided they are not suppressed and complicated by mercury, iodine or other poisonous drugs. We never interfere with the original lesion, but allow Nature to discharge the poisons through the channels established for this purpose.

Under this rational treatment, discharge and ulcer act as fontanels to the system. Not only the specific poison, but much of hereditary and acquired disease matter also are eliminated in the process; and after such a cure, blood and tissues of the patient are purer than they were before infection.

The foregoing statement has nothing to do with the moral aspects involved in acquiring venereal diseases. In this connection we are dealing solely with the rational or irrational treatment of the infection after it has been contracted. We do not wish to intimate that it is advisable to cure the body by killing the soul.

Nevertheless, we must deal with the facts in Nature as we find them. Furthermore, a great many persons, especially women and children, acquire these diseases innocently. Are we not justified in relieving their minds of needless fear and in showing them the way to prevent the dreadful sufferings of the secondary and tertiary stages brought on by suppressive drug treatment by means of mercury, the iodides, "606," etc.?

These poisonous drugs suppress the initial lesion and diffuse the disease poison through the system. Nature takes up the work of elimination by means of skin eruptions and ulcers in various parts of the body, but these also are promptly suppressed with mercurial ointments and other alternatives. This process of suppression is continued for months and years, until the organism is so thoroughly saturated with alterative poisons that vital force can no longer react by acute reactions against the original syphilitic poisons. This state of vital paralysis is then called a cure.

The medical professor, however, knows better. He instructs the students from the lecture platform: "When, after two or three years of mercurial treatment, syphilitic symptoms cease to appear, you may permit the patient to marry—**but never guarantee a cure.**"

Why not? Because the professor is aware that the offspring of such a union are born with hereditary symptoms well known to every physician, and because the patient thus cured (?) may turn up in the doctor's office at any time thereafter with a hole in his palate, ulcers on his body, caries of the bones or with other secondary and tertiary symptoms.

Mercury has an especial affinity for the bony structures. It will work its way through the vertebrae of the spine and the bones of the skull into the nerve matter of the brain and spinal cord, causing inflammation, excruciating headaches, nervous symptoms, girdle pains, etc. These stages of acute inflammation are followed in a few years by sclerosis (hardening) of nerve matter and blood vessels, resulting in paresis, locomotor ataxy or paralysis agitans.

Neither is it necessary to contract specific diseases in order to fall a victim to these dreadful conditions: mercury, iodine and other destructive alternatives are given in a hundred different forms for a multitude of other ailments.

A few years ago we had under our care a patient in the last stages of locomotor ataxy, who for years had been suffering the tortures of the damned. There had never been a taint of specific disease in her system, but four different times in her life she had been salivated by calomel (a common laxative containing mercury). This dreadful poison was given to her in large doses for the cure of liver trouble and constipation. She was only fourteen years old when, on account of this, she first suffered from acute mercurial poisoning.

Another patient who, after fifteen years of slow and torturous dying by inches, succumbed to the same disease, absorbed the mercurial poison in his boyhood days while attending a boarding school. He was twice salivated by mercurial ointments applied to cure the itch (scabies), a disease which was epidemic at times among the boys. He likewise never had a syphilitic disease.

A young man, insane at the age of thirty, absorbed the infernal poison when four years of age. He had at the time a psoric skin eruption, but the family physician suspected syphilitic infection from the nurse girl and kept the child under mercury for six months. How do we know that the diagnosis of syphilis was false? Because the iris of the eye revealed "psora" as the cause of the suspicious eruption which reappeared several times later in life, and because the servant girl was afterwards absolutely exonerated by competent physicians.

Proofs by the Diagnosis from the Eye

We have treated many hundreds of cases of so-called chronic neuralgia, neuritis, rheumatism, neurasthenia, epilepsy and idiocy, due to the pernicious effects of quinine, iodine, arsenic, strychnine, coal-tar products and other virulent poisons taken under the guise of medicine.

How do we know that this is so?

a. Eye Because the Diagnosis from the Eye plainly reveals the presence of these poisons in the system.

b. Because the drug signs in the eye are accompanied by the symptoms of these poisons in the system.

c. Because the record in the eye is confirmed by the history of the patient.

d. Because, under natural living and treatment, diseases long ago suppressed by drugs or knife reappear as healing crises.

e. Because, in these healing crises, drugs indicated by the signs in the iris of the eye are frequently eliminated under their own peculiar symptoms.

f. Because, to the extent that a drug is eliminated from the system by a healing crisis, its sign will disappear from the iris of the eye.

To illustrate:

a. The Diagnosis from the Eye reveals heavy quinine poisoning in the region of the brain.

b. This enables us to say to the patient, without questioning him, that he suffers from severe frontal headaches and ringing in the ears, that he is very irritahle, and so on through the various symptoms of quinine poisoning.

c. The history of the patient reveals the fact that he has taken large amounts of quinine for colds, la grippe or malaria.

d. Under our methods of natural living and treatment, the patient improves; the organism becomes more vigorous, and the organs of elimination act more freely; the latent poisons are stirred up in their hiding places; healing crises make their appearance. The processes of elimination thus inaugurated develop various symptoms of acute poisoning. The eliminating crises are accompanied by headaches, ringing in the ears, nasal catarrh, bone pains, neuritis, strong taste of quinine in the mouth, etc.

e. Every healing crisis, if naturally treated, diminishes the signs of disease and drug poisons in the eye.

Chapter VIII

Inflammation

From what has already been said on this subject, it will have become apparent that inflammatory and feverish diseases are just as natural, orderly and lawful as anything else in Nature, that, therefore, after they have once started, they must not be checked or suppressed by poisonous drugs and surgical operations.

Inflammatory processes can be kept within safe limits, and they must be assisted in their **constructive** tendencies by the natural methods of treatment. To check and suppress acute diseases before they have run their natural course means to suppress Nature's purifying and healing efforts, to court fatal complications and to change the acute, constructive reactions into chronic disease conditions.

Those who have followed the preceding chapters will remember that their general trend has been to prove one of the fundamental principles of Nature Cure philosophy, namely the **Unity of Disease and Cure.**

We claim that **all acute diseases are uniform in their causes, their purpose,** and if conditions are favorable, uniform also in **their progressive development.**

In former chapters I endeavored to prove and to elucidate the unity of acute diseases in regard to their causes and their purpose, the latter not being destructive, but constructive and beneficial. I demonstrated that the microorganisms of disease are not the unmitigated nuisance and evil which they are commonly regarded, but that, like everything else in Nature, they, too, serve a useful purpose. I showed that it depends upon ourselves whether their activity is harmful and destructive, or beneficial: upon our manner of living and of treating acute reactions.

Let us now trace the unity of acute diseases in regard to their general course by a brief examination of the processes of inflammation and their progressive development through five well-defined stages. We shall base our studies on the most advanced works on pathology and bacteriology.

The Story of Inflammation

To me the story of inflammation has been one of the most wonderful revelations of the complex activities of the human organism. More than anything else it confirms to me the fundamental principles of Nature Cure, the fact that Nature is a good healer, not a poor one.

Before inflammation can arise, there must exist an exciting cause in the form of some obstruction or of some agent inimical to health and life. Such excitants of inflammation may be dead cells, blood clots, fragments of bone and other effete matter produced in the system itself or they may be foreign bodies such as particles of dust, soot, stone, iron or other metals, slivers of wood, etc.; again, they may be microorganisms or parasites.

When one or more of these exciting agents of inflammation are present in the tissues of the body in sufficient strength to call forth the reaction and opposition of the healing forces, the microscope will always reveal the following phenomena, slightly varying under different conditions:

The blood rushes to the area of irritation. Owing to this increased blood pressure, the minute arteries and veins in the immediate neighborhood of the excitant dilate and increase in size. The distension of the blood vessels stretches and thereby weakens their walls. Through these the white blood corpuscles squeeze their mobile bodies and work their way through the intervening tissues toward the affected area.

In some mysterious way they seem to sense the exact location of the danger point and hurry toward it in large numbers like soldiers summoned to meet an invading army. This faculty of the white blood corpuscles to apprehend the presence and exact location of the enemy has been ascribed to chemical attraction and is called *chemotaxis*.

The army of defense is made up of the white blood corpuscles or leukocytes and of connective tissue cells which separate themselves from the neighboring tissues. All these wandering cells possess the faculty of absorbing and digesting microbes. They contain certain proteolytic or protein-splitting ferments, by means of which they decompose and digest poisons and hostile microorganisms. On account of their activity as germ destroyers, these cells have been called germ killers or *phagocytes*. In their movements and actions these valiant little warriors act very much like intelligent beings, animated by the qualities of patience, perseverance, courage, foresight and self-sacrifice.

The phagocytes absorb morbid matter, poisons or microorganisms by enveloping them with their own bodies. It is a hand-to-hand fight, and many of the brave little soldiers are destroyed by the poisons and bacteria which they attack and swallow. What we call pus is made up of the bodies of live and dead phagocytes, disease taints and germs, blood serum, broken-down tissues and cells, in short, the debris of the battlefield.

We can now understand how the processes just described produce the well-known cardinal symptoms of inflammation and fever; the redness, heat and swelling due to increased blood pressure, congestion and the accumulation of exudates; the pain due to irritation and to pressure on the nerves. We can also realize how impaired nutrition and the obstruction and destruction in the affected parts and organs will interfere with and inhibit functional activity.

The organism has still other ways and means of defending itself. At the time of bacterial infection, certain germ-killing substances are developed in the blood serum. Science has named these defensive proteins *alexins.* It has also been found that the phagocyte and tissue cells in the neighborhood of the area of irritation produce antipoisons or natural antitoxins, which neutralize the bacterial poisons and kill the microorganisms of disease.

With the Evil, Nature Provides the Cure

Furthermore, the growth and development of bacteria and parasites is inhibited and finally arrested by their own waste products. We have an example of this in the yeast germ, which thrives and multiplies in the presence of sugar in solution. Living on and digesting the sugar, it decomposes the sugar molecules into alcohol and carbonic acid. As the alcohol increases during the process of fermentation, it gradually arrests the development and activity of the yeast cells.

Similar phenomena accompany the activity of disease germs and parasites. They produce certain waste products which gradually inhibit their own growth and increase. The vaccines, serums and antitoxins of medical science are prepared from these bacterial excrements and from extracts made of the bodies of bacteria.

In the serum and antitoxin treatment, therefore, the allopathic school is imitating Nature's procedure in checking the growth of microorganisms, but with this difference: Nature does not suppress the growth and multiplication of disease germs **until the morbid matter on which they subsist has been decomposed and consumed,** and until the inflammatory processes have run their course through the five stages of inflammation; while serums and antitoxins given in powerful doses at the different stages of any disease may check and suppress germ activity and the processes of inflammation before the latter have run their natural course and before the morbid matter has been eliminated.

The Five Stages of Inflammation

What has been said in former chapters confirms my claim that all acute diseases are uniform in their causes and in their purpose. From the foregoing description of inflammation it will have become clear that they are also uniform in their pathological development. The uniformity of acute inflammatory processes becomes still more apparent when we follow them through their five succeeding stages, that is:

Incubation
Aggravation
Destruction
Abatement
Reconstruction

I. Incubation, the time between the exposure to an infectious disease and its development. This period may last from a few minutes to a few days, weeks, months or even years.

During this stage morbid matter, poisons, microorganisms and other excitants of inflammation gather and concentrate in certain parts and organs of the body. When they have accumulated to such an extent as to interfere with the normal functions or to endanger the health and life of the organism, the life forces begin to react to the obstruction or threatening danger by means of the inflammatory processes before described.

II. Aggravation. During the period of **Aggravation** the battle between the phagocytes and Nature's antitoxins on the one hand, and the poisons and microorganisms of disease on the other hand, gradually progresses, accompanied by a corresponding increase of fever and inflammation, until it reaches its climax, marked by the greatest intensity of feverish symptoms.

III. Destruction. This battle between the forces of disease and the healing forces is accompanied by the disintegration of tissues due to the accumulation of exudates, to pus formation, the development of abscesses, boils, fistulas, open sores, etc., and to other morbid changes. It involves the destruction of phagocytes, bacteria, blood vessels, and tissues just as a battle between contending human armies results in loss of life and property.

The stage of **Destruction** ends in crisis, which may be either fatal or beneficial. If the healing forces of the organism are in the ascendancy, and if they are supported by right treatment which tends to build up the blood, increase the vitality and promote elimination, then the poisons and the microorganisms of disease will gradually be overcome, absorbed or eliminated and, by degrees, the tissues will be cleared of the debris of the battlefield.

IV. Abatement. The absorption and elimination of exudates, pus, etc., take place during the period of **abatement.** It is accompanied by a gradual lowering of temperature, pulse rate and the other symptoms of fever and inflammation.

V. Resolution or Reconstruction. When the period of Abatement has run its course and the affected areas have been cleared of the morbid accumulations and obstructions, then, during the fifth stage of inflammation, the work of rebuilding the injured parts and organs begins. More or less destruction has taken place in the cells and tissues, the blood vessels and organs of the areas involved. These must now be reconstructed, and this last stage of the inflammatory process is, therefore, in a way the most important. On the perfect regeneration of the injured parts depends the final effect of the acute disease upon the organism.

If the inflammation has been allowed to run its course through the different stages of acute activity and the final stage of Reconstruction, then **every** acute disease, whatever its name and description may be, will prove beneficial to the organism because morbid matter, foreign bodies, poisons and microorganisms have been eliminated from the system; abnormal and diseased tissues have been broken down and built up again to a purer and more normal condition.

As it were, the acute disease has acted upon the organism like a thunderstorm on the sultry, vitiated summer air. It has cleared the system of impurities and destructive influences, and re-established wholesome, normal conditions. Therefore acute diseases, when treated in harmony with Nature's intent, always prove beneficial.

If, however, through neglect or wrong treatment, the inflammatory processes are not allowed to run their natural course, if they are checked or suppressed by poisonous drugs, the ice bag or surgical operations, or if the disease conditions in the system are so far in the ascendancy that the healing forces cannot react properly, then the constructive forces may lose the battle and the disease may take a fatal ending or develop into chronic ailments.

Suppression During the First Two Stages of Inflammation

It may be suggested that suppression **during the stages of Incubation and Aggravation** need not have fatal consequences if followed by natural living and eliminative treatment. To this I would reply: "Such procedure always involves **the danger of concentrating the disease poisons in vital parts and organs,** thus laying the foundation for chronic destructive diseases."

Furthermore, it is not at all necessary to suppress inflammatory processes by poisonous drugs and other unnatural means, because we can easily and surely control them and keep them from becoming dangerous by our natural means of treatment.

I shall now endeavor to prove and to illustrate the foregoing theoretical expositions by following the development of various diseases through the five stages of inflammation. I shall first take up the commonest of all forms of disease, the cold.

Catching a Cold

According to popular opinion, the catching of colds is responsible for the greater portion of human ailments. Almost daily I hear from patients who come for consultation: All my troubles date back to a cold I took at such and such a time, etc. Then I have to explain that colds are not taken suddenly and from without but that they come **from within,** that their period of Incubation may have extended over months or years, that a clean, healthy body possessed of good vitality **cannot** take cold under the ordinary thermal conditions congenial to human life, no matter how sudden the change in temperature.

At first glance, this may seem to be contrary to common experience as well as to the theory and practice of medical science. But let us follow the development of a cold from start to finish. This will throw some light on the question as to whether it can be caught, or whether it develops slowly within the organism; also whether this development or incubation may extend over a long period of time.

Taking cold may be caused by chilling of the surface of the body or part of the body. In the chilled portions of the skin the pores close, the blood recedes into the interior, and as a result of this the elimination of poisonous gases and exudates through these portions of the skin is suppressed.

This catching a cold through being exposed to a cold draft, through wet clothing, etc., is not necessarily followed by more serious consequences. If the system is not too much encumbered with morbid matter and if kidneys and intestines are in fairly good working order, these organs will take care of the extra amount of waste and morbid materials in place of the temporarily inactive skin and eliminate them without difficulty. The greater the vitality and the more normal the composition of the blood, the better the system will react in such an emergency and throw off the morbid matter which failed to be eliminated through the skin.

If, however, the organism is already overloaded with waste and morbid materials, if the bowels and the kidneys are already weakened and atrophied through continued overwork and overstimulation, if, in addition to this, the vitality has been lowered through excesses or overexertion and the vital fluids are in an abnormal condition, then the morbid matter thrown into the circulation by the chilling and temporary inactivity of the skin cannot find an outlet through the regular channels of elimination and endeavors to escape by way of the mucous linings of the nasal passages, the throat, bronchi, stomach, bowels and genitourinary organs.

The waste materials and poisonous exudates which are being eliminated through these internal membranes cause irritation and congestion, and thus produce the well-known symptoms of inflammation and catarrhal elimination: sneezing (coryza), cough, expectoration, mucous discharges, diarrhea, leucorrhea [vaginal discharge], etc. In other words, these so-called colds are nothing more or less than different forms of vicarious elimination. The membranous linings of the internal organs are doing the work for the inactive, sluggish and atrophied skin, kidneys and intestines. The greater the accumulation of morbid matter in the system, the lower the vitality, and the more abnormal the composition of the blood and lymph, the greater will be the liability to the catching of colds.

What is to be gained by suppressing the different forms of catarrhal elimination with cough and catarrh cures containing opiates, astringents, antiseptics, germkillers and antipyretics? Is it not obvious that such a procedure interferes with Nature's purifying efforts, that it hinders and suppresses the inflammatory processes and the accompanying elimination of morbid matter from the system? Worst of all, that it adds drug poisons to disease poisons?

Such a course can have but one result, namely the changing of Nature's cleansing and healing efforts into chronic disease.

From the foregoing it will have become clear that the cause of a cold lies not so much in the cold draft, or the wet feet, as in **the primary causes of all disease: lowered vitality, deterioration of the vital fluids and the accumulation of morbid matter and poisons in the system.**

The incubation period of the cold may have extended over many years or over an entire lifetime.

What, then, is the **natural cure** for colds? There can be but one remedy: increased elimination through the proper channels. This is accomplished by judicious dieting and fasting, and through restoring the natural activity of the skin, kidneys and bowels by means of wet packs, cold sprays and ablutions, sitz baths, massage, chiropractic or osteopathic manipulation, homeopathic remedies, exercise, sun and air baths and all other methods of natural treatment that save vitality, build up the blood on a normal basis and promote elimination without injuring the organism.

Suppression During the Third Stage of Inflammation

Should the inflammatory processes be suppressed **during the stage of Destruction,** the results would be still more serious and far-reaching. We have learned that during this stage the affected parts and organs are involved in more or less disintegration. They are filled with morbid exudates, pus, etc., which interfere with and make impossible normal nutrition and functioning. If suppression takes place during this stage, it is obvious that the affected areas will be left permanently in a condition of destruction.

Here is an illustration from practical life: Suppose necessary changes and repairs have to be made in a house. Workmen have torn down the partitions, hangings, wallpaper, etc. At this stage of the proceedings the owner discharges the workmen and the house is left in a condition of chaos. Surely, this would not be rational. It would leave the house unfit for habitation. But such a procedure would correspond exactly to the suppression of inflammatory diseases during the stage of Destruction. This also leaves the affected organs permanently in an abnormal, diseased condition.

That accounts for the mysterious sequelae or chronic after-effects which so often follow drug-treated acute diseases. I have traced numerous cases of chronic affections of the lungs and kidneys, of infantile paralysis and of many other chronic ailments to such suppression. In the following I shall describe a typical case, which came under our care and treatment a few years ago.

Suppression by Means of the Ice Bag

A few years ago several gentlemen of Greek nationality called on me with the request that I visit a friend of theirs who had been lying sick for about two months in one of our great West Side [Chicago] hospitals. On investigation I found that the patient had entered the hospital suffering from a mild case of pneumonia. The doctors of the institution had ordered **ice packs.** Rubber sheets filled with ice were applied to the chest and other parts of the body. This had been done for several weeks until the fever subsided.

As a matter of fact, ice is more suppressive than antifever medicines. The continued icy cold applications chill the parts of the body to which they are applied, depress the vital functions and effectually suppress the inflammatory processes.

The result in this case, as in many similar ones which I had occasion to observe during and after the ice-bag treatment, was that the inflammation in the lungs had been arrested and suppressed **during the stage of destruction,** when the air cells and tissues were filled with exudates, blood serum, pus, live and dead blood cells, bacteria, etc., leaving the affected areas of the lungs in a consolidated, liver-like condition.

As a consequence of suppression in the case of this Greek patient, the pneumonia had been changed from the acute to the subacute and chronic stages and the doctors in charge had told his friends that he was now suffering from miliary tuberculosis, and would probably die within a week or two.

After receiving this discouraging information, the friends of the patient came to me and prevailed upon me to take charge of the case. He was transferred to our institution, and we began at once to apply the natural methods of treatment. Instead of ice packs we used the regular cold-water packs, strips of linen wrung out of water of ordinary temperature wrapped around the body and covered with several layers of flannel bandages.

The wet packs became warm on the body in a few minutes. They relaxed the pores and drew the blood into the surface, thus promoting heat radiation and the elimination of morbid matter through the skin.

They did not suppress the fever, but kept it below the danger point.

Under this treatment, accompanied by fasting and judicious osteopathic manipulation, the inflammatory and feverish processes suppressed by the ice packs soon revived, became once more active and aggressive, and were now allowed to run their natural course through the stages of **destruction, absorption** (abatement) and **reconstruction.**

The result of the Nature Cure treatment was that about two months after the patient entered our institution, his friends bought him a ticket to sunny Greece. He had a good journey, and in the congenial climate of his native country made a perfect recovery.

I have observed a number of similar cases suffering from consolidation of the lungs and the resulting asthmatic or tubercular conditions, which had been doctored into these chronic ailments by means of antipyretics and of ice.

Equally dangerous is the ice bag if applied to the inflamed brain or the spinal column. Only too often it results either in paralysis or in death. In many instances, acute cerebrospinal meningitis is changed in this way by drug and serum treatment or by the use of ice bags into the chronic, so-called incurable infantile paralysis.

We say so-called incurable because we have treated **and cured** such cases in all stages of development from the acute inflammatory meningitis to the chronic paralysis of long standing.

In our treatment of acute diseases we never use ice or icy water for packs, compresses, baths or ablutions, but always **water of ordinary temperature** as it comes from the faucet. The water compress or pack warms up quickly, and thus brings about a natural reaction within a few minutes, while the ice bag or pack continually chills and practically freezes the affected parts and organs. This does not allow the skin to relax; it prevents a warm reaction, the radiation of the body heat and the elimination of morbid matter through the skin.

Suppression During the Fourth and Fifth Stages of Inflammation

Let us see what happens when acute diseases are suppressed **during the stages of abatement and reconstruction.** If the defenders of the body, the phagocyte and antitoxins, produced in the tissues and organs, gain the victory over the inimical forces which are threatening the health and life of the organism, then the symptoms of inflammation, swelling, redness, heat, pain and the accelerated heart action which accompanies them, gradually subside. The debris of the battlefield is carried away through the venous circulation which forms the drainage system of the body.

When in this way all morbid materials have been completely eliminated, **Vital Force,** "the physician within," will commence to regenerate and reconstruct the injured and destroyed cells and tissues.

If, however, these processes of elimination and reconstruction are interfered with or interrupted before they are completed, then the affected parts and organs will not have a chance to become entirely well or strong. They will remain in an abnormal, crippled condition, and their functional activity will be seriously handicapped.

The After-effects of Drug-Treated Typhoid Fever

In hundreds of cases I have told patients after a glance into their eyes that they were suffering from chronic indigestion, malassimilation and malnutrition caused by **drug-treated typhoid fever;** and every time the records in the eyes were confirmed by the history of the patient.

In such cases the outer rim of the iris shows a wreath of whitish or drug-colored circular flakes. I have named this wreath "the typhoid rosary." It corresponds to the lymphatic and other absorbent vessels in the intestines, and appears in the iris of the eye when these structures have been injured or atrophied by drug, ice or surgical treatment. Wherever this has been done, the venous and lymphatic vessels in the intestines do not absorb the food materials and these pass through the digestive tract and out of the body without being properly digested and assimilated.

During the destructive stages of typhoid fever, the intestines become denuded by the sloughing of their membranous linings. These sloughed membranes give the stools of the typhoid fever patient their peculiar pea soup appearance. In a similar manner the lymphatic, venous and glandular structures which constitute the absorbent vessels of the intestines atrophy and slough away.

If the inflammatory processes are allowed to run their normal course under natural methods of treatment through the stages of Destruction, Absorption and Reconstruction, Nature will rebuild the membranous and glandular structures of the intestinal canal perfectly, convalescence will be rapid and the patient will enjoy better health than before he contracted the disease.

If, however, through injudicious feeding or the administration of quinine, mercury, purging salts, opiates or other destructive agents, Nature's processes are interfered with, prematurely checked and suppressed, then the sloughed membranes and absorbent vessels are not reconstructed, and the intestinal tract is left in a denuded and atrophied condition.

Such a patient may arise from his bed thinking that he is cured; but unless he is afterward treated by natural methods, he will never make a full recovery. It will take him, perhaps, months or years to die a gradual, miserable death through malassimilation and malnutrition, which usually end in some form of wasting disease, such as pernicious anemia or tuberculosis. If he does not actually die from the effects of the wrongly treated typhoid fever, he will be troubled all his life with intestinal indigestion, constipation, malassimilation and the accompanying nervous disorders.

A Change for the Better

Speaking of typhoid fever, we are glad to say that for this particular form of disease the most advanced medical science has adopted the Nature Cure treatment, that is, **straight cold water and fasting,** and **no drugs,** as it was originated by the pioneers of Nature Cure in Germany more than fifty years ago.

This treatment, which medical science has found so eminently successful in typhoid fever, would prove equally efficacious in all other acute diseases if the regular doctors would only try it. It is a strange and curious fact that so far they have never found it worth while to do so. All Nature Cure physicians know from their daily experience in actual practice that **the simple water treatment and fasting is sufficient to cure all other forms of acute diseases just as easily and effectively as typhoid fever.** By this is proved the **unity of treatment** in all acute diseases.

Both in typhoid fever and in tuberculosis, progressive medical men have now entirely abandoned the germ-killing method of treatment. They have found it absolutely useless and superfluous to hunt for drugs and serums to kill the typhoid and tuberculosis bacilli in these, the two most destructive diseases afflicting the human family. They were forced to admit that the simple remedies of the Nature Cure school, cold water and fasting in typhoid fever and the fresh-air treatment in tuberculosis, are the only worthwhile methods to fight these formidable enemies to health and life.

If they would continue their researches and experiments along

these **natural** lines, they would attain infinitely more satisfactory results than through their germ-hunting and germ-killing theories and
practices.

CHAPTER IX

The Effects of Suppression of Venereal Diseases

Another good illustration of suppression may be found in the allopathic treatment of venereal diseases. Almost invariably the drug treatment suppresses these diseases in the stages of **incubation** and **aggravation,** thus locking them up in the system. The venereal taints and germs, however, are living things which grow and multiply until the body has been completely permeated by them. Then they must find an outlet somehow and somewhere, and consequently they break out in the manifold so-called "secondary" and "tertiary" symptoms.

The drug poisons which are used to "cure" (suppress) these symptoms, greatly aggravate the disease. They create conditions in the system infinitely worse than the venereal diseases themselves. Thus the acute, easily curable stages of these ailments are changed into the dreadful and obstinate chronic conditions. It is in this way that venereal diseases are made hereditary and transmitted to future generations.

In a special article on this subject entitled "Venereal Diseases," published in *"The Naturopath,"* January, 1913, 1 have substantiated the following claims:

1. "Venereal diseases are not necessarily chronic in their progressive development.

2. "They are essentially acute and self-limited. But **may become chronic** through neglect or through suppressive drug treatment.

3. "The chronic, so-called secondary and tertiary manifestations of venereal diseases, such as ulceration of bones and fleshy tissue, gummata of the brain, sclerosis of the spinal cord, arthritic rheumatism, degeneration and destruction of other vital parts and organs of the body, are not so much the result of the original gonorrheal or syphilitic infection, as of the destructive drug poisons which have been taken to cure or rather to suppress the primary lesions and acute inflammatory symptoms.

4. "Venereal diseases in the acute inflammatory stages are easily and completely curable by natural methods of living and of treatment.

5. "Venereal diseases treated and cured by natural methods **during the acute inflammatory stages** are never followed by any chronic after-effects or secondary and tertiary manifestations whatsoever.

6. "When venereal diseases have reached the secondary and tertiary stages, they are still curable by natural methods of living and of treatment, providing there is left sufficient vitality to respond to treatment and providing the destruction of vital parts and organs has not advanced too far.

"Hundreds of cases of well-developed locomotor ataxy, paresis, and other so-called secondary and tertiary diseases of the brain and the nervous system, of bony and fleshy tissues, and of vital organs have been cured by our natural methods of treatment.

"It is self-evident, however, that the treatment and cure of the chronic conditions require more patience and perseverance than the cure of acute conditions not tampered with and suppressed by drugs.

7. "Venereal diseases treated and cured by natural methods are never followed by chronic after-effects. On the other hand, mercury, iodine, quinine, and coal-tar poisons produce all the so-called secondary and tertiary symptoms of syphilis in people who never in their lives were afflicted with venereal diseases, but who have taken or absorbed these drug poisons in other ways.

". . . These facts are proven beyond doubt by the Diagnosis from the Eye. All, destructive poisons taken in sufficient quantities will in time reveal their presence and exact location in the body through certain well-defined signs or discolorations in the iris.

"These poisons undermine the structures of the body and deteriorate vital parts and organs so slowly and insidiously that the superficial observer does not trace and connect cause and effect."

The Wasserman and Noguchi Tests

Medical men may say to the foregoing that the Wasserman and Noguchi tests furnish positive proofs of syphilis in the system. These chemical tests are supposed to reveal with certainty the presence of venereal taints in the body,—at least, the public is left under this impression.

I am convinced, however, that in many instances the "positive" Wasserman or Noguchi tests are the result of mercurial poison instead of syphilitic infection. In a number of cases where these tests proved "positive," that is, where, according to the theory of allopathic medical science, they indicated a luetic condition of the system, the subjects of these tests had never in their lives shown any symptoms of syphilis nor, as far as they knew, had they ever been exposed to infection, but every one of them showed plainly the sign of mercurial poisoning in the iris of the eye, and had taken considerable mercury in the form of calomel or of other medicinal preparations for diseases **not of a luetic nature,** or they had been "salivated" by coming in contact with the mercurial poison in mines, smelters, mirror factories, etc.

This leads me to believe that, sooner or later, medical science will have to admit that the Wasserman and Noguchi tests reveal, in many instances at least, the effects of mercurial poisoning instead of the effects of syphilitic infection. And this would not be surprising since it is well known that mercury has very similar effects upon the system as syphilis.

It takes the mercurial poison from five to ten and even fifteen years before it works its way into the brain and spinal cord, and there causes its characteristic degeneration and destruction of brain and. nerve tissues which manifest outwardly as locomotor ataxy, paralysis agitans, paresis, apoplexy, hemiplegia, epilepsy, St. Vitus dance, and the different forms of idiocy and insanity. Mercurial poisoning is also in many instances the cause of deafness and blindness.

When the symptoms of mercurial destruction begin to show, then they, in turn, are suppressed by preparations of iodine, the "606," or other "alteratives," and so the merry war goes, on: poison against poison, Beelzebub against the Devil, and the poor suffering body has to stand it all.

In this way the system is periodically saturated with the most virulent poisons on earth, until the undertaker finishes the job. And this is miscalled "scientific treatment." There never was invented by cruel Indian or fanatical inquisition worse torture than this. They mercifully finished the sufferings of their victims within a few hours or, at the worst, days; but this torture inflicted upon human beings in the name of medical science continues for a lifetime. It means dying by inches under the most horrible conditions for ten, twenty, thirty years or longer.

In this connection it may be well to quote the testimony of Professor E. A. Farrington of Philadelphia, one of the most celebrated homeopathic physicians of the nineteenth century. He says, in his *"Clinical Materia Medica,"* third edition, page 141:

"The various constitutions or dyscrasia underlying chronic and acute affections are, indeed, very numerous. As yet, we do not know them all. We do know that one of them comes in gonorrhoea, a disease which is frightfully common, so that the constitution arising from this disease is rapidly on the increase.

"Now I want to tell you why it is so. It is because allopathic physicians, and many homeopaths as well, do not properly cure it. I do not believe gonorrhoea to be a local disease. If it is not properly cured, a constitutional poison which may be transmitted to the children is developed. I know, from years of experience and observation, that gonorrhoea is a serious difficulty, and one, too, that complicates many cases that we have to treat.

"The same is true of syphilis in a modified degree. Gonorrhoea seems to attack the nobler tissues, the lungs, the heart, and the nervous system, all of which are reached by syphilis only after the lapse of years."

The Destructive After-Effects of Mercury

Concerning the destructive after-effects of mercury, of which homeopaths have made a most careful study, Professor Farrington says, on pages 558-559 of the same volume:

"The more remote symptoms of mercurial poisoning are these: You will find that the blood becomes impoverished. The albumin and fibrin of that fluid are affected. They are diminished, and you find in their place a certain fatty substance, the composition of which I do not exactly know. Consequently, as a prominent symptom, the body wastes and emaciates. The patient suffers from fever which is rather hectic in its character. The periosteum becomes affected, and you then have a characteristic group of mercurial pains, bone pains worse in changes of the weather, worse in the warmth of the bed, and chilliness with or after stool. The skin becomes rather of a brownish hue; ulcers form, particularly on the legs; they are stubborn and will not heal. The patient is troubled with sleeplessness and ebullitions of blood at night; he is hot and cannot sleep; he is thrown quickly into a perspiration, which perspiration gives him no relief.

"The entire system suffers also, and you have here two series of symptoms. At first the patient becomes anxious and restless and cannot remain quiet; he changes his position; he moves about from place to place; he seems to have a great deal of anxiety about the heart, praecordial anguish, as it is termed, particularly at night.

"Then, in another series of symptoms, there are jerkings of the limbs, making the patient appear as though he were attacked by St. Vitus' dance. Or, you may notice what is more common yet, trembling of the hands, this tremor being altogether beyond the control of the patient and gradually spreading over the entire body, giving you a resemblance to paralysis agitans or shaking palsy.

"Finally, the patient becomes paralyzed, cannot move his limbs, his mind becomes lost, and he presents a perfect picture of imbecility. He does all sorts of queer things. He sits in the corner with an idiotic smile on his face, playing with straws; he is forgetful, he cannot remember even the most ordinary events. He becomes disgustingly filthy and eats his own excrement. In fact, he is a perfect idiot.

"Be careful how you give mercury; it is a treacherous medicine. It seems often indicated. You give it and relieve; but your patient is worse again in a few weeks and then you give it again with relief. By and by, it fails you. Now, if I want to make a permanent cure, for instance, in a scrofulous child, I will very seldom give him mercury; should I do so, it will be at least only as an intercurrent remedy."

Chapter X

Suppressive Surgical Treatment of
Tonsillitis and Enlarged Adenoids

The following paragraphs are taken from an article in the *Nature Cure Magazine* May, 1909, titled "Surgery for Tonsillitis and Adenoids." They will throw further interesting light on the dangerous consequences of suppressing acute and subacute diseases.

"The tonsils are excreting glands. Nature has created them for the elimination of impurities from the body. Acute, subacute and chronic tonsillitis accompanied by enlargement and cheesy decay of the tonsils means that these glands have been habitually congested with morbid matter and poisons, that they have had more work to do than they could properly attend to.

"**These glandular structures constitute a valuable part of the drainage system of the organism.** If the blood is poisoned through overeating and faulty food combinations, or with scrofulous, venereal or psoriatic poisons, the tonsils are called upon, along with other organs, to eliminate these morbid taints. Is it any wonder that frequently they become inflamed and subject to decay? What, however, can be gained by destroying them with iodine or extirpating them with the surgeon's scissors or the 'guillotine'?

"Because your servants are weakened by overwork, would you kill them? Because the drains in your house are too small to carry off the waste, would you blockade or remove them? Still, this is the orthodox philosophy of the medical schools applied to the management of the human body.

". . . In case of any morbid discharge from the body, wherever it be, whether through hemorrhoids, open sores, ulcers or through tonsils, scrofulous glands, etc., a fontanelle has been established to which and through which systemic poisons make their way. If such an outlet be blocked by medical or surgical treatment the stream of morbid matter has to seek another escape or else the poisons will accumulate somewhere in the body.

"Fortunate is the patient when such an escape can be established, because wherever in the system morbid excretions, suppressed by medical treatment, concentrate, there will inevitably be found the seat of chronic disease.

"After the tonsils have been removed, the morbid matter which they were eliminating usually finds the nearest and easiest outlet through the adenoid tissues and nasal membranes. These now take up the work of 'vicarious' elimination and, in their turn, become hyperactive and inflamed.

"Sometimes it happens that the adenoid tissues become affected **before** the tonsils. In that case, also, relief through the surgeon's knife is sought and then the process is reversed: after the adenoids have been removed, the tonsils develop chronic catarrhal conditions.

"When both tonsils and adenoids have been removed, the nasal membranes will, in turn, become congested and swollen. Often the mucous elimination increases to an alarming degree, and frequently polyps and other growths make their appearance or the turbinated bones soften and swell and obstruct the nasal passages, thus **again making the patient a 'mouth breather.'**

"But in vain does Nature protest against local symptomatic treatment. Science has nothing to learn from her.

"When the nose takes up the work of vicarious elimination, the same mode of treatment is resorted to. The mucous membranes of the nose are now swabbed and sprayed with antiseptics and astringents, or 'burned' by cauterizers, electricity, etc. The polyps are cut out, and frequently parts of the turbinated bone and septum as well, in order to open the air passages.

"Now, surely, the patient must be cured. But, strange to say, new and more serious troubles arise. The posterior nasal passages and the throat are now affected by chronic catarrhal conditions and there is much annoyance from phlegm and mucous discharges which drop into the throat. These catarrhal conditions frequently extend to the mucous membranes of stomach and intestines.

"When the drainage system of the nose and the nasopharyngeal cavities has been completely destroyed, the impurities must either travel upward into the brain or downward into the glandular structures of the neck, thence into the bronchi and the tissues of the lungs.

"If the trend be upward, to the brain, the patient grows nervous and irritable or becomes dull and apathetic. How often is a child reprimanded or even punished for laziness and inattention when it cannot help itself? In many instances the morbid matter affects certain centers in the brain and causes nervous conditions, hysteria, St. Vitus' dance, epilepsy, etc. In children the impurities frequently find an outlet through the eardrums in the form of pus-like discharges. This may frequently avert inflammation of the brain, meningitis, imbecility, insanity or infantile paralysis.

"If the trend of the suppressed impurities and poisons be downward, it often results in the hypertrophy and degeneration of the lymphatic glands of the neck. In such cases the suppressive treatment, by drugs or knife, is again applied instead of eliminative and curative measures. The scrofulous poisons, suppressed and driven back from the diseased glands in the neck, now find lodgment in the bronchi and lungs, where they accumulate and form a luxuriant soil for the growth of the bacilli of pneumonia and tuberculosis.

"In other cases, the vocal organs become seriously affected by chronic catarrhal conditions, abnormal growths and in later stages by tuberculosis. Many a fine voice has been ruined in this way.

"The prevention and the cure of all these ailments lie not in local symptomatic treatment and suppression by drugs or knife, but in the rational and natural treatment of the body as a whole."

Chapter XI

Cancer

Let us see how our theories of the Unity of Disease and Cure apply to cancer, the much-dreaded and rapidly increasing disease which is considered absolutely incurable by both the laity and the medical profession.

Allopathy says that the only possible remedy is "early operation." Nevertheless, in the textbooks of medical science and in medical schools and colleges it is taught that cancer and all other malignant growths **"always return after extirpation."** In fact, every student of medicine is expected to state this in his examination papers as part of the definition of malignant tumors.

The great majority of medical practitioners hold, furthermore, that cancer is a **local** disease. This is proved by the fact that they apply local, symptomatic treatment.

In reality, however, the disease is **constitutional.** Therefore, after removal of the growth by surgery, the electric needle, X-Rays, etc., the cancer or tumor is liable to break out again in the same place or in several places.

The surest way to change insignificant, so-called "benign" (not fatal to life) fibroid or fatty tumors into malignant cancer or sarcoma is to operate upon them. Wens and warts are often made malignant by surgical interference or other local irritation.

In my article titled "What We Know About Cancer" in the August, 1909, issue of the *Nature Cure Magazine* I quote from an article by Burton J. Hendrick, the cancer expert, published in the July, 1909, number of *McClure's Magazine,* as follows:

> "Clinical observation long ago established the fact that any irritating interference with a cancer almost always stimulates its growth. In his earliest experiments Dr. Loeb found that, by merely drawing a silk thread through a dormant or slowly developing tumor, he could transform it into a rapidly growing one. Cutting with a knife produced the same effect. This accounts for the commonly observed fact that, when extirpated cancers in human beings recur, they increase in size much more rapidly than the original growth."

The late Dr. Senn, the great cancer surgeon, admitted these facts in an interview given to Chicago press representatives upon his return from his trip around the world in 1906. The press clipping reads as follows.

"Avoid Beauty Doctors"

"Incidentally, Dr. Senn advises women who worry over their disfigurement of moles about their heads and shoulders to have those so-called beauty spots removed early in life, but he tells them they should not go to beauty doctors to have the operations performed.

"He knows of hundreds of cases, he says, where cancer has resulted from the irritation of moles by an electric needle, or by constant picking it. 'Have a surgeon cut the mole out,' is his advice, as it will hurt little and leave no scar."

To this we answered in our comments on the interview: "If the little knife of the beauty doctor causes cancer, what about the big knife of the surgeon?"

In point of fact, our office records show that a large percentage of malignant growths are the direct result of surgical operations.

Cancer Not a Local, But a Constitutional Disease

For many years I have been teaching in my lectures and writings as well as in private advice to patients that cancer is a constitutional disease; that it is rooted in every drop of blood in the body; that it is caused by the presence of certain disease taints or of food and drug poisons in the system; that these poisons irritate and stimulate the cells in a certain locality and cause their abnormal multiplication or proliferation in the forms of benign or malignant tumors.

I also claim that meat eating has much to do with the causation of cancer.

Certain discoveries by Dr. H. C. Ross of London, England, confirm my claims that cancer is not at all of local and accidental origin, but that **it is constitutional,** and that it may be caused by the gradual accumulation in the system of certain poisons which form in decaying animal matter.

One day, while experimenting in his laboratory, Dr. Ross brought white blood cells or leucocytes into contact with a certain aniline dye on the slide of a microscope and noticed that they began at once to multiply by cell division (proliferation). This was the first time that cell proliferation had been observed by the human eye while the cells were separated from their parent organism.

Dr. Ross realized that he had made an important discovery and continued his experiments under the microscope in order to find out what other substances would cause cell multiplication. He found that certain xanthines and albuminoids derived from decaying animal matter were the most effective for this purpose and induced more rapid cell proliferation than any other substances he was able to procure.

Dr. Ross obtained these "alkaloids of putrefaction," as he called them, from blood which had been allowed to putrefy in a warm place. He found that albuminoids derived from decaying **vegetable** substances did not have the same effect.

His discoveries led him to believe that the alkaloids of putrefaction produced in a cut or wound by the decaying of dead blood and tissue cells are the cause of the rapid multiplication of the neighboring live cells, which gradually fill the wound with new tissues.

Thus, for the first time in the history of medicine, a rational explanation of Nature's methods for repairing injured tissues has been advanced.

Dr. Ross applied his theory still farther to the causation of benign and malignant growths, reasoning that the alkaloids of putrefaction produced in or attracted to a certain part of the body by some local irritation are the cause of the rapid, abnormal multiplication of cells in tumor formations.

In benign tumors the abnormal proliferation of cells takes place slowly, and they do not tend to immediate and rapid decay and deterioration.

In malignant tumors the "wild" cells, created in immense numbers, decay almost as rapidly as they are produced because the abnormal growths are devoid of normal organization. They have no established, regular blood and nerve supply, nor are they provided with adequate venous drainage. They are, therefore, cut off from the orderly life of the organism and doomed to rapid deterioration.

The processes of decay of these tumor materials liberate large quantities of alkaloids of putrefaction, and these, in turn, stimulate the normal, healthy cells with which they come in contact to rapid, abnormal multiplication.

The malignant growth, therefore, feeds on its own products of decay, aside from the systemic poisons and morbid materials already contained in the blood and tissues of the body. These morbid products permeate the entire system. They are carried by the circulation of the blood into all parts of the body. This explains why cancer is a constitutional disease, why it is, as I stated it, "rooted in every drop of blood."

It also explains why cancer, or rather the disposition to its development (diathesis), is hereditary.

If the original cancerous growth is removed by surgical intervention, X-Rays, the electric needle, cauterization or any other form of local treatment, the poisonous materials (alkaloids of putrefaction) in the blood will set up other foci of abnormal, wild proliferation. Medical science has applied the term metastasis to such spreading and reappearing of malignant tumors after extirpation.

Dr. Ross' findings throw an interesting light on the relationship between cancer and meat eating. Is it not self-evident that in a digestive tract filled most of the time with large masses of partially digested and decaying animal food enormous quantities of alkaloids of putrefaction are created? These are absorbed into the circulation, attracted to any point where exists some form of local irritation and then stimulate the cells in that locality to abnormal proliferation.

"But," it will be said, "meat eating alone does not account for cancer, because vegetarians also succumb to the disease." This is true. Alkaloids of putrefaction are constantly produced in every animal and human body. They form in the excretions of living cells and in the decaying protoplasm of dead cells, and if the organs of elimination do not function properly, these morbid materials will accumulate in the system.

Furthermore, the Diagnosis from the Eye furnishes positive proof that Hahnemann's **theory of psora** is based on truth. I quote from my article in the *Nature Cure Magazine* August, 1909:

> "For a hundred years, Hahnemann's theory of psora has been scouted and ridiculed by the allopathic schools and even among homeopaths only a few have accepted it. Now we are confronted by the remarkable fact that, at this late day, the Diagnosis from the Eye confirms the observations and speculations of the great genius of homeopathy.
> "After suppression of itchy eruptions, lice, crab lice, etc., spots ranging in color from light brown to dark red appear in different places in the iris of the eye. These 'itch spots' indicate the organs and localities of the body in which the suppressed disease taints have concentrated.

"Such suppressions represent not only the scrofulous taints which Nature was trying to eliminate by means of eruptions and parasites, but, in addition to these, the poisons contained in the bodies of the parasites and the drug poisons which were used to suppress or kill them.

"It has been found that the bodies of the itch parasites (*Sarcoptes scabici*) contain an exceedingly poisonous substance which the homeopaths call 'psorinum'. When these minute animals burrowing in and under the skin are killed by poisonous drugs and antiseptics, the morbid taints in their bodies are absorbed by the system and added to the psoriatic poisons which Nature has been trying to eliminate.

"Thus, after suppression of itchy eruptions or parasites, the organism is encumbered with three poisons instead of one: (1) the hereditary or acquired scrofulous and psoriatic taints which the cells of the body were throwing off into the blood stream and which the blood was feeding to the parasites on the surface, (2) the morbid substance contained in the bodies of the parasites, (3) the drug poisons used as suppressants. (Such poisons may lie latent in the system for many years before they become active and, in combination with other disease taints and with food and drug poisons, create the different forms of chronic destructive diseases.)

"These facts explain why the itch spots in different areas of the iris of the eye so frequently indicate serious chronic, destructive disease conditions in the parts and organs of the body corresponding to these areas, why; for instance, in asthma and tuberculosis we often find itch spots in the region representing the lungs or why in cancer of the liver or of the stomach itch spots show in the area of stomach or liver.

"That the itch or psoriatic taint is actually at the bottom of the cancerous diathesis is attested by the fact that all cancer patients whom we have treated and cured, with two exceptions (whose healing crisis took the form of furunculosis), broke out with the itch at one time or another during the natural treatment. In most of these cases the bodies of the patients were inflamed with fiery eruptions for days or even weeks at a time.

"Nature Cure allows these healing crises to run their course unhindered and unchecked; in fact, we encourage them by air and sun baths, cold-water treatment and homeopathic remedies."

What has been said verifies my claim that benign and malignant tumors can be cured only by thorough purifying the system of all morbid and poisonous taints and by building up the blood to a normal basis, that is, by providing it with the proper elements of nutrition, especially with the all-important organic salts.

That this is not merely theory, but actual fact has been proved in the great cancer institutes in Europe and in this country. The scientists in charge of these institutions report that they have found a positive cure for cancer in animals. The treatment is as follows:

The blood is pumped out of the body of a dog or other animal afflicted with cancer and immediately afterwards the blood of a healthy animal which has shown immunity to cancer inoculation is pumped into the body of the diseased animal. It is reported that in nine cases out of ten thus treated the cancerous growths disappear.

This treatment, of course, entails the death of the animal which had to give up its life blood to cure the other and therefore this method of cure is not adaptable to human beings. Even though an individual, with suicidal intent, would be willing to give up his life for a stipulated legacy to his relatives, the law would not sanction the transaction.

However, we of the Nature Cure school say that it is not necessary to pump the diseased blood out of the organism. In the natural methods of living and of treatment we possess the means of **purifying and regenerating that blood while it is in the body.** That this is possible we have proved in a number of cancer cases.

It is obvious, however, that the earlier the disease is treated by the natural methods, that is, before the breaking-down process has far advanced, the easier and quicker will be the cure.

In the case of tumors, then, we see again verified the fundamental law of Nature Cure: the Unity of Disease and of Treatment. We see that the tumor is not of local, but of constitutional, origin, that its period of incubation may extend over a lifetime or over several generations.

Chapter XII

Women's Suffering

Certain ailments peculiar to the female organism have become almost universal among civilized races. Probably the majority of surgical operations are performed for so-called women's diseases. That women suffer untold agonies during menstruation, in childbirth and at the climacteric is looked upon as unavoidable and a matter of course.

The fact that the native women of Africa, of the Sandwich Islands, the South American bush and our western plains are practically exempt from these ailments indicates that the cause of female troubles must lie in artificial habits of living and in the unnatural treatment of diseases.

Many are beginning to recognize these truths. For them is dawning a new era, when knowledge will free Woman from physical suffering as it has freed her from other bondage.

Instances like the following are of common occurrence in our free clinics for Diagnosis from the Eye:

A lady tells us that she has been suffering for many years from a complication of female troubles. Her eyes show a heavy scurf rim, indicating an inactive, atrophied skin, poor surface circulation and, as a result of this condition, defective elimination through the skin and accumulation of waste matter and systemic poisons in the system. The areas of stomach and intestines reveal the signs of chronic catarrhal affection and atrophy of the membranous linings and glandular structures. This, of course, means indigestion, fermentation of foods, gas formation, constipation and a multitude of resulting disturbances.

The signs in the iris also indicate an atonic, relaxed and prolapsed condition of stomach, bowels and other abdominal organs. This is likely to cause sagging of the genital organs, relaxation of the bands and ligaments which hold them in place and, as a result of this relaxation, misplacement of the womb.

We tell the patient of our findings in her eyes and she admits all the conditions and symptoms which we describe, but she is not satisfied because our diagnosis does not agree with that of the great specialists and professors of medicine whom she has consulted. Every one of them has told her that all her troubles are due to the fact that her uterus is flexed and retroverted, that it presses on the rectum (this being the cause of her chronic constipation and of the obstructed menstrual flow, the congestion, pain, etc.), and **that the womb must be placed in its normal position by a surgical operation.**

In this and many similar cases that have come to us for treatment, it was the relaxed and prolapsed condition of the stomach and intestines that caused the sinking (prolapsus) of the uterus with the attending distressing symptoms. In some instances the womb and with it the bladder had fallen so low that they protruded from the vagina. In all of these cases, as the patients without exception told us, the professors and specialists assured them that surgical treatment, shortening of the ligaments, the insertion of pessaries, the cutting loose and raising of the womb, etc., were the only possible means of curing these ailments.

So we explain to the lady that the relaxed and prolapsed condition of the genital organs, the misplacement of the womb, etc., are **not** causes of disease, but only the effects of the weakened and relaxed condition of the digestive organs, and that this, in turn, is due to indigestion, malnutrition, defective elimination through skin, bowels and kidneys; that, therefore, the only possibility of cure lies in correcting and overcoming these constitutional conditions through an eliminative diet, blood-building remedies and other natural methods; that the blood must be built up on a normal basis, and that the digestive tract and the other abdominal organs must be made more alive and active through hydropathic treatment, massage, spinal manipulation, general and special exercises, air and sun baths, etc.

In thousands of cases we have thus cured female troubles without poisonous drugs or surgical operations, simply by improving the digestion, purifying the blood and invigorating the abdominal organs in a natural manner.

On the other hand, almost daily we meet with instances of untold suffering as the direct consequence of operations, the use of pessaries, etc., which only served to weaken the genital organs still more and resulted in all sorts of complications, inflammations, adhesions, etc., and in many cases in malignant tumors.

In this connection I would warn especially against the use of pessaries. They are at best only a mechanical contrivance, and do not add anything to the improvement of the diseased condition. On the other hand, they irritate the abdominal organs by excessive pressure, which in many instances produces inflammation of the neighboring tissues and abnormal growths.

Suppressing inflammation of the genital organs by poisonous antiseptics, sprays, tampons or other local applications only tends to aggravate the chronic conditions. Curetting (scraping) the womb does not cure the catarrhal affection, but only serves to destroy its delicate mucous lining and to suppress catarrhal elimination. Holding up the womb by means of a pessary in order to strengthen its muscles and ligaments is about as reasonable and effective as to try to strengthen a weak arm by carrying it in a sling. Replacing or removing misplaced or affected organs by means of surgery does not contribute anything toward correcting the causes of these abnormal conditions, but in many instances makes a real cure impossible. How can an organ be cured after it has been extirpated with the knife?

It is a fact known to every observing physician that from fifty to seventy-five percent of all women have some kind of misplacement of the genital organs and that only a comparatively small number of these suffer from local disturbances, indicating that, in most cases, misplacement alone will not create serious trouble.

It is ridiculous to assume that the small, flabby uterus of an anemic woman can block the rectum and cause disease, but it is an excellent talking point, as effective in bringing victims to the operating table as appendicitis with its fairy tales of seeds and foreign bodies lodging in the appendix vermiformis.

While studying Nature Cure in Germany, I took special courses in the Thure-Brandt Massage. By means of this internal manipulative treatment, weakness of ligaments and muscles, displacements, adhesions, etc., can be corrected without the use of knife or drugs. During my first years in practice, I frequently resorted to the internal manual treatment with good results; but I found that in most cases it was not at all necessary in order to produce perfect cures.

I saw that chiropractic and osteopathic correction of spinal and pelvic lesions and consequent removal of irritation and pressure on the nerves, the cure of chronic constipation and malnutrition by pure food diet and hydrotherapy, the strengthening of the pelvic muscles and nerves by means of active and passive movements and exercises, were fully sufficient to correct the local symptoms in a natural manner. Thousands of cases cured by us by these methods attest the truth of our statements; while those who failed to understand the simple reasoning of the Nature Cure philosophy or lacked will power to withstand the arguments of friends and physicians followed the siren call of the operating table and have been sorry for it ever since.

In case of operation for misplacement of the womb, it is necessary, in order to keep the womb in its new position, to stitch it to the frontal abdominal wall. Very frequently it will not stay there, breaks loose, and relapses into an abnormal position. Granted that it remains fixed, woe to the woman if she becomes pregnant. The womb cannot assume the constantly changing positions of pregnancy, and the result is either abortion or malformation of the fetus, together with great and constant suffering to the woman.

The operation has done nothing to correct unnatural habits of living or to purify the system of its scrofulous and psoriatic taints, of drug and food poisons. Frequently these gather in the parts that have been weakened and irritated by the antiseptics and by the surgeon's knife, and set up new inflammations, ulcerations and only too often malignant tumors. As a result, one operation follows another.

We cannot cut in the genital organs without cutting in the brain. The nervous system is a unit, and the brain is directly and intimately connected with the complex and highly sensitive nerve centers of the genital organs. Mutilation of the genital nerve centers, therefore, invariably affects the brain, and thus the intellectual and emotional life of a woman. It is almost axiomatic that a woman whose uterus or ovaries have been removed or mutilated is afterward mentally and emotionally more or less abnormal. Nervousness, irritability and only too often nervous prostration and insanity are the sequelae of operative treatment.

In medical colleges, among students and professors, these facts are freely admitted and discussed, but the prospective patient hears a different story. "Cut loose the womb, shorten the ligaments, put it into the right position, and everything will be well." This sounds plausible and seductive; but everyday experiences expose the inadequacy and the destructive aftereffects of local symptomatic treatment.

The Climacteric or Change of Life

Under our artificial methods of living, the *climacteric* or change of life, has become the bugbear of womanhood. It seems to be universally assumed that this period in a woman's life must be fraught with manifold sufferings and dangers. It is taken as a matter of course that during these changes in her organism a woman is assailed by the most serious physical, mental, and psychic ailments which may endanger her sanity and often her life.

Like rheumatism, neurasthenia, neuralgia and hundreds of other medical terms, "change of life" is a convenient phrase to cover the doctor's ignorance. No matter what ailments befall a woman during the years from forty to fifty, may the causes be ever so obscure, the diagnosis is easy. "You are in the climacteric, you are suffering from the change of life," says the doctor, and the patient is satisfied and resigns herself to the inevitable.

Frequently women come to us for consultation, and after reciting a long string of troubles they conclude with the remark: "Of course, doctor, I'm in the change, and I know that lots of these things are **natural** at my time of life."

Is it true that all this suffering is natural and inevitable?Among the primitive races of the earth suffering incident to the change of life is practically unknown. The same is true in a lesser degree of the country population of Europe. The causes of it must, therefore, be sought in the artificial modes of living peculiar to our hypercivilization and in the unnatural methods of treating disease as commonly practiced.

Which are the specific causes of the profound disturbances so often accompanying the organic changes of the climacteric?

Aside from their other physiological functions, the menses are for the woman a monthly cleansing crisis through which Nature eliminates from her system considerable amounts of waste and morbid matter which, under a natural regime of life, would be discharged by means of the organs of depuration, that is, the lungs, skin, kidneys and bowels.

The more natural the life and the more normal, as the result of this, the woman's physical condition, the shorter and less annoying and painful, within certain limits, will be the menstrual periods.

Through unnatural habits of eating, drinking, dressing, breathing and through equally unnatural methods of medical treatment, the kidneys, skin and bowels have become inactive, benumbed or paralyzed. As long as the vicarious monthly purification by means of the menses continues, the evil results of the torpid condition of the regular organs of depuration do not become so apparent. The organism has learned to adapt itself to this mode of elimination.

But when, on account of the organic changes of the climacteric, menstruation ceases, then the systemic poisons, which formerly were eliminated by means of this monthly purification, accumulate in the system and become the source of all manner of trouble. All tendencies to physical, mental or psychic disease are greatly intensified. The poisonous taints circulating in the blood overstimulate or else depress and paralyze the brain and the nervous system. As a consequence, mental and psychic disorders are of common occurrence; the more so because the waning of the sex functions is accompanied by a tendency to negativity and hypersensitiveness.

How Can the Ailments of the Climacteric Be Avoided or Cured?

Is it not self-evident that the easiest way to sidestep the troubles incident to this critical period and to reestablish the perfect equilibrium of the organism lies in restoring the natural activity of the organs of elimination?

This is what Nature Cure accomplishes easily and successfully with its natural methods of treatment. Air and sun baths, water treatments and massage bring new life and activity to the enervated skin. Pure food diet, chiropractic and osteopathic treatment, curative gymnastics, homeopathic or herb remedies restore the natural tonicity and functioning of the stomach, liver, kidneys and intestines. Mental therapeutics, systematically practiced, make every cell in the body vibrant with the higher and finer forces of the mental and spiritual planes of being.

When the natural equilibrium of the organism is thus restored, there is absolutely no occasion for the troubles of the climacteric. We have proved this in hundreds of cases. As kidneys, skin and bowels begin to function normally and freely, physical and mental conditions commence to improve, and one after another the dreaded symptoms disappear.

Let us compare with this common sense, natural treatment the orthodox medical practice in such cases:

The medical treatment, as usual, is entirely symptomatic. The sluggish organs of elimination are prodded by poisonous cathartics, laxatives, diaphoretics, cholagogues and tonics, all of which, after temporary stimulation, leave the organs in a more weakened and the system in a more poisoned condition. If brain and nerves are irritated and aching, sedatives and hypnotics are given to stupefy them into insensibility. If the heart action is weak and irregular, it is whipped up by poisonous stimulants; if too fast, it is checked and paralyzed by sedatives and depressants.

Thus, instead of removing the underlying causes, every symptom is promptly suppressed. Drug poisons are added to the waste and morbid matter which are already clogging the channels of life. And, of course, under such unnatural treatment, in many instances things go from bad to worse. Flushes, headaches, rheumatic and neuralgic pains, melancholia, irritability, mental aberration, partial paralysis and a multitude of other symptoms appear and gradually increase in severity.

When the family physician has arrived at the end of his wits, the surgeon has his innings, and leaves the patient in a still worse condition of chronic suffering.

These experiences are so common that the manifold troubles of the climacteric are regarded as unavoidable and as a matter of course. Here, as in so many other instances, people fail to see that it is the treatment which prevents the cure. If the efficiency of common sense, natural treatment were more widely known and recognized, how much unnecessary suffering could be avoided.

Chapter XIII

The Treatment of Acute Diseases by Natural Methods

In the preceding chapters we have described the results of the wrong, that is, **suppressive** treatment of acute diseases. We shall now proceed to describe the simple and uniform methods of natural treatment.

If the uniformity of acute diseases be a fact in Nature, then it follows that **it must be possible to treat all acute diseases by uniform methods.**

That it is possible to treat **all** acute diseases most successfully by natural methods, which anybody possessed of ordinary intelligence can apply, has been demonstrated for more than seventy years by the Nature Cure practitioners in Germany, and by myself during the last ten years in an extensive practice.

One of the many advantages of natural treatment is that it may be applied right from the beginning, as soon as the first symptoms of acute febrile conditions manifest themselves. It is not necessary to wait for a correct diagnosis of the case.

The regular physician, with his specific treatment for the multitude of specific diseases which he recognizes, often has to wait several days or even weeks before the real nature of the disease becomes clear to him, before he is able to diagnose the case or even to make a good guess. The conscientious medical practitioner has to postpone actual treatment until the symptoms are well defined. Meanwhile he applies expectant treatment as it is called in medical parlance, that is, he gives a purgative or a placebo, something or other to placate, or to make the patient and his friends believe that something is being done.

But during this period of indecision and inaction very often the best opportunity for aiding Nature in her healing efforts is lost, and the inflammatory processes may reach such virulence that it becomes very difficult or even impossible to keep them within constructive limits. The bonfire that was to burn up the rubbish on the premises may, if not watched and tended, assume such proportions that it damages or destroys the house.

It must also be borne in mind that very frequently acute diseases do not present the well-defined sets of symptoms which fit into the accepted medical conception of certain specific ailments. On the contrary, in many instances the symptoms suggest a combination of different forms of acute diseases.

If the character of the disease is ill-defined and complicated, how, then, is the physician of the "Old School" to select the proper specific remedy, Under such circumstances, the diagnosis of the case as well as the medical treatment will at best be largely guesswork.

Compare with this unreliable and unsatisfactory treatment the simple and scientific, exact and efficient natural methods. **The natural remedies can be applied from the first,** at the slightest manifestation of inflammatory and febrile symptoms. No matter what the specific nature or trend of the inflammatory process, whether it be a simple cold, or whether it take the form of measles, scarlet fever, diphtheria, smallpox, appendicitis, etc.—it makes absolutely no difference in the mode of treatment. In many instances the natural treatment will have broken the virulence of the attack or brought about a cure before the regular physician gets good and ready to apply his specific treatment.

In the following I shall describe briefly these natural methods for the treatment of acute diseases which insure the largest possible percentage of recoveries and at the same time do not in any way tax the system, cause undesirable aftereffects or lead to the different forms of chronic invalidism.

The Natural Remedies

The most important ones of these natural remedies can be had free of cost in any home. They are: air, fasting or eliminative diets, water, and the right mental attitude.

I am fully convinced that these remedies offered freely by Mother Nature are sufficient, if rightly applied, to cure any acute disease arising within the organism. If circumstances permit, however, we may advantageously add corrective manipulation of the spine, massage, magnetic treatment, advanced regenerative modalities (like the Magnatherm) and homeopathic, herbal and specific nutritional supplementation.

The Fresh-Air Treatment

A plentiful supply of pure fresh air is of vital importance at any time. We can live without food for several weeks and without water for several days, but we cannot live without air for more than a few minutes. Just as a fire in the furnace cannot be kept up without a good draft which supplies the necessary amount of oxygen to the flame, so the fires of life in the body cannot be maintained without an abundance of oxygen in the air we breathe.

This is of vital importance at all times, but especially so in acute disease, because here, as we have learned, all the vital processes are intensified. The system is working under high pressure. Large quantities of waste and morbid materials, the products of inflammation, have to be oxidized, that is, burned up and eliminated from the system.

In this respect the Nature Cure people have brought about one of the greatest reforms in medical treatment: the admission of plenty of fresh air to the sickroom.

But, strange to say, the importance of this most essential natural remedy is as yet not universally recognized by the representatives of the regular school of medicine. Time and again I have been called to sickrooms where by order of the doctor every window was closed and the room filled with pestilential odors, the poisonous exhalations of the diseased organism added to the stale air of the unventilated and often overheated apartment. And this air starvation had been enforced by graduates of our best medical schools and colleges. This unnatural and inexcusable crime against the sick is committed even at this late day in our great hospitals under the direct supervision of physicians who are foremost in their profession.

It is not the cold draft that is to be feared in the sickroom. Cool air is most agreeable and beneficial to the body burning in fever heat. **What is to be feared is the reinhalation and reabsorption of poisonous emanations from the lungs and skin of the diseased body.**

Furthermore, the ventilation of a room can be so regulated as to provide a constant and plentiful supply of fresh air without exposing its occupants to a direct draft. Where there is only one window and one door, both may be opened and a sheet or blanket hung across the opening of the door, or the single window may be opened partly from above and partly from below, which insures the entrance of fresh, cold air at the bottom and the expulsion of the heated and vitiated air at the top. The patient may be protected by a screen, or a board may be placed across the lower part of the window in such manner that a direct current of air upon the patient is prevented.

In very cold weather, or if conditions are not favorable to constant ventilation of the sickroom, the doors and windows may be opened **wide** for several minutes every few hours, while the patient's body and head are well protected. There is absolutely no danger of taking cold if these precautions are taken. Under right conditions of room temperature, frequent exposure of the patient's nude body to air and the sunlight will be found most beneficial and will often induce sleep when other means fail.

I would strongly warn against keeping the patient **too warm.** This is especially dangerous in the case of young children, who cannot use their own judgment or make their wishes known. I have frequently found children in high fever smothered in heavy blankets under the mistaken impression on the part of the attendants that they had to be kept warm and protected against possible draft. In many instances the air under the covers was actually steaming hot. This surely does not tend to reduce the burning fever heat in the body of the patient.

"Natural Diet" in Acute Diseases

From the appearance of the first suspicious symptoms until the fever has abated and there is a hearty, natural hunger, feeding should be reduced to a minimum or better still, entirely suspended.

In cases of extreme weakness, and where the acute and subacute processes are long drawn out and the patient has become greatly emaciated, it is advisable to give such easily digestible foods as white of egg, milk, buttermilk and whole grain bread with butter in combination with raw and stewed fruits and with vegetable salads prepared with lemon juice and olive oil.

The quantity of drinking water should be regulated by the desire of the patient, but he should be warned not to take any more than is necessary to satisfy his thirst. Large amounts of water taken into the system dilute the blood and the other fluids and secretions of the organism to an excessive degree, and this tends to increase the general weakness and lower the patient's resistance to the disease forces.

Water may be made more palatable and at the same time more effective for purposes of elimination by the addition of the unsweetened juice of acid fruits, such as orange, grapefruit or lemon, about one part of juice to three parts of water. Fresh pineapple juice is very good except in cases of hyperacidity of the stomach. The fresh, unsweetened juice of Concord grapes is also beneficial.

Acid and subacid fruit juices do not contain sufficient carbohydrate or protein materials to unduly excite the digestive processes, while on the other hand they are very rich in **Nature's best medicines, the mineral salts in organic form.** Sweet grapes and sweetened grape juice should not be given to patients suffering from acute, febrile diseases because they contain too much sugar, which would have a tendency to start the processes of digestion and assimilation, to cause morbid fermentation and to raise the temperature and accelerate the other disease symptoms.

Fasting

Total abstinence from food during acute febrile conditions is of primary importance. In certain diseases which will be mentioned later on, especially those involving the digestive tract, fasting must be continued for several days after all fever symptoms have disappeared.

There is no greater fallacy than that the patient must be sustained and his strength kept up by plenty of nourishing food and drink or, worse still, by stimulants and tonics. This is altogether wrong in itself, and besides, habit and appetite are often mistaken for hunger.

A common spectacle witnessed at the bedside of the sick is that of well-meaning but misguided relatives and friends **forcing** food and drink on the patient, often by order of the doctor, when his whole system rebels against it and the nauseated stomach expels the food as soon as taken. Sedatives and tonics are then resorted to in order to force the digestive organs into submission.

Aversion to eating during acute diseases, whether they represent healing crises or disease crises, is perfectly natural, because the entire organism, including the mucous membranes of stomach and intestines, is engaged in the work of **elimination, not assimilation.** Nausea, slimy and fetid discharges, constipation alternating with diarrhea, etc., indicate that the organs of digestion are throwing off disease matter, and that they are not in a condition to take up and assimilate food.

Ordinarily, the digestive tract acts like a sponge which absorbs the elements of nutrition; but in acute diseases the process is reversed, the sponge is being squeezed and gives off large quantities of morbid matter. The processes of digestion and assimilation are at a standstill. In fact, the entire organism is in a condition of prostration, weakness and inactivity. The vital energies are concentrated on the cleansing and healing processes. Accordingly, there is no demand for food.

This is verified by the fact that a person fasting for a certain period, say, four weeks, during the course of a serious acute illness, will not lose nearly as much in weight as the same person fasting four weeks in days of healthful activity.

It is for the foregoing reasons that nourishment taken during acute disease:

1. is not properly digested, assimilated and transmuted into healthy blood and tissues. Instead, it ferments and decays, filling the system with waste matter and noxious gases.

2. interferes seriously with the elimination of morbid matter through stomach and intestines by forcing these organs to take up the work of digestion and assimilation.

3. diverts the vital forces from their combat against the disease conditions and draws upon them to remove the worse than useless food ballast from the organism.

This explains why taking food during feverish diseases is usually followed by a rise in temperature and by aggravation of the other disease symptoms. As long as there are signs of inflammatory, febrile conditions and no appetite, do not be afraid to withhold food entirely, if necessary, for as long as five, six or seven weeks. In my practice I have had several patients who did not take any food, except water to which acid fruit juices had been added, for more than seven weeks, and then made a rapid and complete recovery.

In cases of gastritis, appendicitis, peritonitis, dysentery or typhoid fever, abstinence from food is absolutely imperative. Not even milk should be taken until fever and inflammation have entirely subsided, and then a few days should be allowed for the healing and restoring of the injured tissues. Many of the serious chronic aftereffects of these diseases are due to too early feeding, which does not allow the healing forces of Nature time to rebuild sloughed membranes and injured organs.

After a prolonged fast, great care must be observed when commencing to eat. Very small quantities of light food may safely be taken at intervals of a few hours. A good plan, especially after an attack of typhoid fever or dysentery, is to break the fast by thoroughly masticating one or two tablespoonfuls of popcorn. This gives the digestive tract a good scouring and starts the peristaltic action of the bowels better than any other food.

The popcorn may advantageously be followed in about two hours with a tablespoonful of cooked rice and one or two cooked prunes or a small quantity of some other stewed fruit.

For several days or weeks after a fast, according to the severity of the acute disease or healing crisis, **a diet consisting largely of raw fruits,** such as oranges, grapefruit, apples, pears, grapes, etc., and juicy vegetables, especially lettuce, celery, cabbage slaw, water-cress, young onions, tomatoes or cucumbers should be adhered to. No condiments or dressings should be used with the vegetables except lemon juice and olive oil.

Hydropathic Treatment in Acute Diseases

We claim that in acute diseases hydropathic treatment will accomplish all the benefcial effects which the "Old School" practitioners ascribe to drugs, and that water applications will produce the desired results much more efficiently, and without any harmful by-effects or aftereffects upon the system.

The principal objects to be attained in the treatment of acute inflammatory diseases are:

1. To relieve the inner congestion and consequent pain in the affected parts.

2. To keep the temperature below the danger point by promoting heat radiation through the skin.

3. To increase the activity of the organs of elimination and thus to facilitate the removal of morbid materials from the system.

4. To increase the positive electromagnetic energies in the organism.

5. To increase the amount of oxygen and ozone in the system and thereby to promote the oxidation and combustion of effete matter.

The above-mentioned objects can be attained most effectually by the simple cold water treatment. Whatever the acute condition may be, whether an ordinary cold or the most serious type of febrile disease, the applications described in detail in the following pages, used singly, combined or alternately according to individual conditions, will always be in order and sufficient to produce the best possible results.

Baths and Ablutions

Cooling sprays or, if the patient is too weak to leave the bed, cold sponge baths or ablutions, repeated whenever the temperature rises, are very effective for keeping the fever below the danger point, for relieving the congestion in the interior of the body and for stimulating the elimination of systemic poisons through the skin.

However, care must be taken not to lower the temperature too much by the excessive coldness or unduly prolonged dura-

tion of the application. It is possible to suppress inflammatory processes by means of cold water or ice bags just as easily as with poisonous antiseptics, antifever medicines and surgical operations.

It is sufficient to reduce the temperature to just below the danger point. This will allow the inflammatory processes to run their natural course through the five progressive stages of inflammation and this natural course will then be followed by perfect regeneration of the affected parts.

In our sanitarium we use only water of ordinary temperature as it flows from the faucet, never under any circumstances ice bags or ice water. The application of ice keeps the parts to which it is applied in a chilled condition. The circulation cannot react, and the inflammatory processes are thus most effectually suppressed.

To recapitulate: **Never check or suppress a fever** by means of cold baths, ablutions, wet packs, etc., **but merely lower it below the danger point.** For instance, if a certain type of fever has a tendency to rise to 104° F. or more, bring it down to about 102°. If the fever ordinarily runs at a lower temperature, say at 102° F., do not try to reduce it more than one or two degrees.

If the temperature is subnormal, that is, below the normal or regular body temperature, the packs should be applied in such a manner that a warming effect is produced, that is, less wet cloths and more dry covering should be used, and the packs left on the body a longer time before they are renewed. More detailed instruction will be given in subsequent pages.

Never lose sight of the fact that fever is in itself a healing, cleansing process which must not be checked or suppressed.

Hot-Water Applications Are Injurious

Altogether wrong is the application of hot water to seats of inflammation as, for instance, the inflamed appendix or ovaries, sprains, bruises, etc. Almost in every instance where I am called in to attend a case of acute appendicitis or peritonitis, I find hot compresses or hot water bottles, by means of which the inflamed parts are kept continually in an overheated condition. It is in this way that a simple inflammation is nurtured into an abscess and made more serious and dangerous.

The hot compress or hot-water bottle draws the blood away from the inflamed area to the surface **temporarily;** but unless the hot application is kept up continually, the blood, under the Law of Action and

Reaction, will recede from the surface into the interior, and as a result the inner congestion will become as great as or greater than before.

If the hot applications are continued, **the applied heat tends to maintain and increase the heat in the inflamed parts.**

Inflammation means that there is already too much heat in the affected part or organ. Common sense, therefore, would dictate cooling applications instead of heating ones.

The cold packs and compresses, on the other hand, have a directly cooling effect upon the seat of inflammation and in accordance with the Law of Action and Reaction **their secondary, lasting effect consists in drawing the blood from the congested and heated interior** to the surface, thus relaxing the pores of the skin and promoting the radiation of heat and the elimination of impurities.

Both the hot-water applications and the use of ice are, therefore, to be absolutely condemned. The only rational and natural treatment of inflammatory conditions is that by compresses, packs and ablutions, using water of ordinary temperature, as it comes from the cold water tap.

By means of the simple cold-water treatment and fasting all fevers and inflammations can be reduced in a perfectly natural way within a short time without undue strain on the organism.

The Whole-Body Pack

The whole-body pack is most effective if by means of it the patient can be brought into a state of copious perspiration. The pack is then removed and the patient is given a cold sponge bath.

It will be found that this treatment often produces a second profuse sweat which is very beneficial. This aftersweat should also be followed by a cold sponge bath.

Such a course of treatment will frequently be sufficient to eliminate the morbid matter which has gathered in the system, and thus prevent in a perfectly natural manner a threatening disease which otherwise might become dangerous to life.

How to Apply the Whole-Body Pack

On a bed or cot spread two or more blankets, according to their weight. Over the top blanket spread a linen or cotton sheet which has been dipped into cold water and wrung out fairly dry. Let the blankets extend about one foot beyond the wet sheet at the head of the bed.

Place the patient on the wet sheet so that it comes well up to the neck, and wrap the sheet snugly around the body so that it covers every part, tucking it in between the arms and sides and between the legs. It will be found that the sheet can be adjusted more snugly and smoothly if separate strips of wet linen are **placed between the legs and between the arms and the sides of the body.**

The blankets are now folded, one by one, upward over the feet and around the body, turned in at the neck and brought across the chest, the outer layers being held in place with safety pins.

The patient should stay in this whole-body pack from one-half hour to two hours, according to the object to be attained and the reaction of the body to the pack. If the pack has been correctly applied, the patient will become warm in a few minutes.

The Bed-Sweat Bath

If the patient does not react to the pack, that is, if he remains cold, or if, as is sometimes the case in malaria, the fever is accompanied by chills or if profuse perspiration is desired, bottles filled with hot water or bricks heated in the oven and wrapped in flannel should be placed along the sides and to the feet, under the outside covering.

This form of application is called the bed-sweat bath. It may be used with good results when an incipient cold is to be aborted.

After the pack has been removed, the body should be sponged with cold water, as already stated. Use a coarse cloth or Turkish towel for this purpose rather than a sponge, as the latter cannot be kept perfectly clean. Dry the body quickly but thoroughly, and finish by rubbing with the hands.

In the meantime the damp bed clothing should be replaced by dry sheets and blankets (a second cot or bed will be found a great convenience), and the patient put to bed without delay and well covered in order to prevent chilling and also to induce, if possible, a copious aftersweat. The patient is then sponged off a second time, put into a dry bed, and allowed to rest.

If the patient is too weak to leave his bed, the cold sponge may be given on a large rubber sheet or oilcloth covered with an old blanket, which should be placed on the bed before the pack is applied. After removing the pack, put a blanket over the patient to prevent chilling and wash quickly but thoroughly first the limbs, then chest and stomach, then the back, drying and covering each part as soon as finished. Remove the rubber sheet from the bed and wrap the patient in dry, warm blankets, or lift him into another bed.

How to Apply the Short-Body Pack

A wide strip of linen or muslin, wrung out of cold water, is wrapped around the patient from under the armpits to the thighs or knees in one, two or more layers, covered by one or more layers of dry flannel or muslin in such a manner that the wet linen does not protrude at any place.

Similar packs may be applied to the throat,* the arms, legs, shoulder joints or any other part of the body.

The number of layers of wet linen and dry covering is determined by the vitality of the patient, the height of his temperature and the particular object of the application, which may be:

1. to lower high temperature

2. to raise the temperature when subnormal

3. to relieve inner congestion

4. to promote elimination.

If the object is to lower high temperature, several layers of wet linen should be wrapped around the body and covered **loosely** by one or two layers of the dry wrappings in order to prevent the bed from getting wet. The packs must be renewed as soon as they become dry or uncomfortably hot.

If the object is to raise subnormal temperature, less wet linen and more dry covering must be used, and the packs left on a longer time, say from thirty minutes to two hours. If the patient does not react to the pack, hot bricks or bottles filled with hot water should be placed at the sides and to the feet, as explained in connection with the whole-body pack.

If inner congestion is to be relieved, or if the object is to promote elimination, less of the wet linen and more dry wrappings should be used.

When packs are applied, the bed may be protected by spreading an oilcloth over the mattress under the sheet. But in no case should oilcloth or rubber sheeting be used for the outer covering of packs. This would interfere with some of the main objects of the pack treatment, especially with heat radiation. The outer covering should be warm but at the same time porous, to allow the escape of heat and of poisonous gases from the body.

Local Compresses

In case of local inflammation, as in appendicitis, ovaritis, colitis, etc., separate cooling compresses may be slipped under the pack and over the seat of inflammation. These local compresses may be removed and changed when hot and dry without disturbing the larger pack.

In all fevers accompanied by high temperature, it is advisable to place an extra cooling compress at the nape of the neck (the region of the medulla and the back brain), because here are located the brain centers which regulate the inner temperature of the body (thermotaxic centers), and the cooling of these brain centers produces a cooling effect upon the entire organism.

Enemas

While ordinarily we do not favor the giving of injections or enemas unless they are absolutely necessary, we apply them freely in feverish diseases in order to remove from the rectum and lower colon any accumulations of morbid matter, and thus to prevent their reabsorption into the system. In cases of exceptionally stubborn constipation, an injection of a few ounces of warm olive oil may be given. Allow this to remain in the colon about thirty minutes in order to soften the contents of the rectum, and follow with an injection of warm water.

Just How the Cold Packs Produce Their Wonderful Results

(1) How Cold Packs Promote Heat Radiation

Many people are under the impression that the packs reduce the fever temperature so quickly because they are put on cold. But this is not so, because, unless the reaction be bad, the packs become warm after a few minutes' contact with the body.

The prompt reduction of temperature takes place because of increased heat radiation. The coldness of the pack may lower the surface temperature slightly; but it is the moist warmth forming under the pack on the surface of the body that draws the blood from the congested interior into the skin, relaxes and opens its minute blood vessels and pores, and in that way facilitates the escape of heat from the body.

In febrile conditions the pores and capillary blood vessels of the skin are tense and contracted. Therefore the heat cannot escape, the skin is hot and dry, and the interior of the body remains overheated.

When the skin relaxes and the patient begins to perspire freely, we say the fever is broken.

The moist warmth under the wet pack produces this relaxation of the skin in a perfectly natural manner. By means of these simple packs followed by cold ablutions, the temperature of the patient can be kept at any point desired without the use of poisonous antifever medicines, serums and antitoxins which lower the temperature by benumbing and paralyzing heart action, respiration, the red and white blood corpuscles, and thus generally lowering the vital activities of the organism.

(2) How Cold Packs Relieve Inner Congestion

In all inflammatory febrile diseases the blood is congested in the inflamed parts and organs. This produces the four cardinal symptoms of inflammation: redness, swelling, heat, and pain. [Rubor, tumor, colar and dolar.] If the congestion be too great, the pain becomes excessive, and the inflammatory processes cannot run their natural course to the best advantage. It is therefore of great importance to relieve the local blood pressure in the affected parts and this can be accomplished most effectively by means of the wet packs.

As before stated, **they draw the blood onto the surface of the body and in that way relieve inner congestion wherever it may exist,** whether it be in the brain, as in meningitis, in the lungs, as in pneumonia, or in the inflamed appendix.

In several cases where a child was in the most dangerous stage of diphtheria, where the membranes in throat and nasal passages were already choking the little patient, the wet packs applied to the entire body from neck to feet relieved the congestion in the throat so quickly that within half an hour after the first application the patient breathed easily and soon made a perfect recovery. The effectiveness of these simple water applications in reducing congestion, heat and pain is little short of marvelous.

(3) How Cold Packs Promote Elimination

By far the largest number of deaths in febrile diseases result from the accumulation in the system of poisonous substances, which paralyze or destroy vital centers and organs. Therefore it is necessary to eliminate the morbid products of inflammation from the organism as quickly as possible.

This also is accomplished most effectively and thoroughly by the application of wet packs. As they draw the blood into the surface and relax the minute blood vessels in the skin, **the morbid materials in the**

blood are eliminated through the pores of the skin and absorbed by the packs. That this is actually so is verified by the yellowish or brownish discoloration of the wet wrappings and by their offensive odor.

One of the main causes of constipation in febrile diseases is the inner congestion and fever heat. Through the cooling and relaxing effect of the packs upon the intestines, this inner fever heat is reduced, and a natural movement of the bowels greatly facilitated.

If constipation should persist in spite of the packs and cooling compresses, injections of tepid water should be given every day or every other day in order to prevent the reabsorption of poisonous products from the lower colon. **But never give injections of cold water with the idea of reducing fever in that way.** This is very dangerous and may cause fatal collapse.

The Electromagnetic Effect of Cold Water Applications

One of the most important, but least understood, effects of hydropathic treatment is its influence upon the electromagnetic energies in the human body. At least, I have never found any allusions to this aspect of the cold-water treatment in any books on hydrotherapy which have come to my notice.

The sudden application of cold water or cold air to the surface of the nude body and the inhalation of cold air into the lungs have the effect of increasing the amount of electromagnetic energy in the system.

This can be verified by the following experiment: Insert one of the plates of an electrometer (sensitive galvanometer) into the stomach of a person who has remained for some time in a warm room. Now let this person inhale suddenly **fresh, cold outside air.** At once the galvanometer will register a larger amount of electromagnetic energy.

The same effect will be produced by the application of a quick, cold spray to the warm body.

It is the sudden lowering of temperature on the surface of the body or in the lungs and the resulting contrast between the heat within and the cold outside, that causes the increased manifestation of electromagnetic energy in the system.

This, together with the acceleration of the entire circulation, undoubtedly accounts for the tonic effect of cold-water applications such as cold packs, ablutions, sprays, sitz baths, barefoot walking, etc., and for the wonderfully bracing influence of fresh, cold outside air.

The energizing effect of cold air may also explain to a large extent the superiority of the races inhabiting the temperate zones over those of the warm and torrid southern regions.

To me it seems a very foolish custom to run away from the invigorating northern winters to the enervating sameness of southern climates. One of the reasons I abandoned, with considerable financial sacrifice, a well-established home in a Texas city which is the Mecca of health-seekers, was that I did not want to rear my children under the enervating influence of that beautiful climate. I, for my part, want some cold winter weather every year to stir up the lazy blood corpuscles, to set the blood bounding through the system and to freeze out the microbes.

In our Nature Cure work we find all the way through that the continued application of warmth has a debilitating effect upon the organism, and that only by the opposing influences of alternating heat and cold can we produce the natural stimulation which awakens the dormant vital energies in the body of the chronic.

Increase of Oxygen and Ozone

The liberation of electromagnetic currents through cold-water applications has other very important effects upon the system besides that of stimulation.

Electricity splits up molecules of water into hydrogen, oxygen and ozone. We have an example of this in the thunderstorm. The powerful electric discharges which we call lightning separate or split the watery vapors in the air into these elements. It is the increase of oxygen and ozone in the air that purifies and sweetens the atmosphere after the storm.

In acute as well as in chronic disease, large amounts of oxygen and ozone are required to burn up the morbid materials and to purify the system. Certain combinations of these elements are among the most powerful antiseptics and germicides.

Likewise, the electric currents produced by cold packs, ablutions and other cold-water applications split up the molecules of water in the tissues of the body into their component parts. In this way large amounts of oxygen and ozone are liberated, and these elements assist to a considerable extent in the oxidation and neutralization of waste materials and disease products.

The following experiment proves that sudden changes in temperature create electric currents in metals: When two cylinders of dissimilar metals are welded together, and one of the metals is suddenly chilled or heated, electric currents are produced which will continue to flow until both metals are at the same temperature.

Another application of this principle is furnished by the oxydonor. If both poles of this little instrument are exposed to the same temperature, there is no manifestation of electricity; but if one of the poles be attached to the warm body and the other immersed in cold water or exposed to cold air, the liberation of electromagnetic currents begins at once. These electric currents set free oxygen and ozone, which in their turn support the oxidation and neutralization of systemic poisons.

According to my experience, however, the cold-water applications are more effective in this respect than the oxydonor.

The Importance of Right Mental and Emotional Attitude in Acute Disease

We have learned that in the processes of inflammation a battle is going on between the healing forces of the body, the phagocytes and natural antitoxins on the one hand and the disease taints, germs, bacilli, etc., on the other hand.

This battle is real in every respect, as real as a combat between armies of living soldiers. In this conflict, going on in all acute inflammatory diseases, mind plays the same role as the commander of an army.

The great general needs courage, equanimity and presence of mind most in the stress of battle. So the mind, the commander of the vast armies of cells battling in acute disease for the health of the body, must have absolute faith in the superiority of Nature's healing forces.

If the mind becomes frightened by the inflammatory and febrile symptoms and pictures to itself in darkest colors their dreadful consequences, these confused and distracted thought vibrations are conveyed instantaneously to the millions of little soldiers fighting in the affected parts and organs. They also become confused and panic-stricken.

The excitement of fear in the mind still more accelerates heart action and respiration, intensifies the local congestion and greatly increases the morbid accumulations in the system. In the last chapters of this volume we shall deal especially with the deteriorating influence of fear, anxiety, anger, irritability, impatience, etc., and explain how these and all other destructive emotions actually poison the secretions of the body.

In acute disease we cannot afford to add to the poisonous elements in the organism, because the danger of a fatal ending lies largely in the paralysis of vital centers by the morbid and poisonous products of inflammation.

Everything depends upon the maintenance of the greatest possible inflow of vital force; and there is nothing so weakening as worry and anxiety, nothing that impedes the inflow, distribution and normal activity of the vital energies like fear. A person overcome by sudden fright is actually benumbed and paralyzed, unable to think and to act intelligently.

These truths may be expressed in another way. The victory of the healing forces in acute disease depends upon an abundant supply of the positive electromagnetie energies. In the initial chapters of this volume we have learned that health is positive, disease negative. The positive mental attitude of faith and equanimity creates positive electromagnetic energies in the body, thus infusing the battling phagocytes with increased vigor and favoring the secretion of the antitoxins and antibodies, while the negative, fearful and worrying attitude of mind creates in the system the negative conditions of weakness, lowered resistance and actual paralysis.

In the paragraphs dealing with the effects of cold-water treatment upon the body we learned that the electric currents created in the organism split up the molecules of water in the tissues into their component elements (hydrogen and oxygen), thus liberating large amounts of oxygen and ozone; and that these, in turn, support the processes of combustion and oxidation in the system, burn up waste and morbid matter, and destroy hostile microorganisms.

However, the electromagnetic forces in the body are not only increased and intensified by positive foods, exercise, cold-water treatment, air baths, etc., but **also by the positive attitude of mind and will.**

The positive mind and will are to the body what the magneto is to the automobile. As the electric sparks from the magneto ignite the gas, thus generating the power that drives the machine, so the positive vibrations, generated by a confident and determined will, create in the body the positive electromagnetic currents which incite and stimulate all vital activities.

Common experience teaches us that the concentration of the will on the thing to be accomplished greatly heightens and increases all physical, mental and moral powers.

Therefore the victory in acute diseases is conditioned by the absolute faith, confidence and serenity of mind on the part of the patient. The more he exercises these harmonizing and invigorating qualities of mind and soul, the more favorable are the conditions for the little soldiers who are fighting his battles in the inflamed parts and organs. The blood and nerve currents are less impeded and disturbed, and flow more normally. The local congestion is relieved, and this favors the natural course of the inflammatory processes.

Therefore, instead of being overcome with fear and anxiety, as most people are under such circumstances, do not become alarmed, nor convey alarm to the millions of little cells battling in the inflamed parts. Speak to them like a commander addressing his troops: "We understand the laws of disease and cure, we know that these inflammatory and febrile symptoms are the result of Nature's healing efforts, we have perfect confidence in her wisdom and in the efficiency of her healing forces. This fever is merely a good house-cleaning, a healing crisis. We are eliminating morbid matter, poisons and germs which were endangering health and life.

"We rejoice over the purification and regeneration now taking place and benefiting the whole body. Fear not! Attend to your work quietly and serenely! Let us open ourselves wide to the inflow of life from the source of all life in the innermost parts of our being! The life in us is the life of God. We are strengthened and made whole by the Divine life and power which animate the universe."

The serenity of your mind, backed by absolute trust in the Law and by the power of a strong Will, infuses the cells and tissues with new life and vigor, enabling them to turn the acute disease into a beneficial, cleansing and healing crisis.

In the following we give a similar formula for treating chronic constipation.

Say to the cells in the liver, the pancreas and the intestinal tract:

> "I am not going to force you any longer with drugs or enemas to do your duty. From now on you must work on your own initiative. Your secretions will become more abundant. Every day at—o'clock the bowels will move freely and easily."

At the appointed time make the effort, whether you are successful or not, and do not resort to the enema until it becomes an absolute necessity. If you combine with the mental and physical effort a natural diet, cold sitz baths, massage and osteopathic treatment, you will have need of the enema at increasingly longer intervals, and soon be able to discard it altogether.

Be careful, however, not to employ your intelligence and your will power to **suppress** acute inflammatory and febrile processes and symptoms. This can be accomplished by the power of the will as well as by ice bags and poisonous drugs, and its effect would be to turn Nature's acute cleansing efforts into chronic disease.

The Importance of Right Mental and Emotional Attitude on the Part of Friends and Relatives

What has just been said about the patient is true also of his friends and relatives. Disease is negative. The sick person is exceedingly sensitive to his surroundings. He is easily influenced by all depressing, discordant and jarring conditions. He catches the expressions of fear and anxiety in the looks, the words, gestures and actions of his attendants, relatives and friends and these intensify his own depression and gloomy forebodings.

This applies especially to the influence exerted by the mother upon her ailing infant. There exists a most intimate sympathetic and telepathic connection between mother and child. The child is affected not only by the outward expression of the mother's fear and anxiety, but likewise by the hidden doubt and despair in the mother's mind and soul.

Usually, the first thing that confronts me when I am called to the sickbed of a child is the frantic and almost hysterical mental condition of the mother, and to begin with, I have to explain to her the destructive influence of her behavior. I ask her:

"Would you willingly give some deadly poison to your child?" "Certainly not," she says, to which I reply:

"Do you realize that you are doing this very thing? That your fear and worry vibrations actually poison and paralyze the vital energies in the body of your child and most seriously interfere with Nature's healing processes?

"Instead of helping the **disease** forces to destroy your child, assist the **healing** forces to save it by maintaining an attitude of absolute faith, serenity, calmness and cheerfulness. Then your looks, your voice, your touch will convey to your child the positive, magnetic vibrations of health and of strength. Your very presence will radiate healing power."

Then I explain how faith, calmness and cheerfulness on her part will soothe and harmonize the discordant disease vibrations in the child's body.

Herein lies the modus operandi or working basis of all successful mental and metaphysical treatment.

Summary

Natural Methods in the Treatment of Acute Disease

I. Fresh Air

A. A plentiful supply of pure air in the sickroom.

B. Frequent exposure of the nude body to air and sun light.

C. Patient must not be kept too warm.

II. Natural Diet

A. The minimum amount of light food, chiefly fruit and vegetable salads, no condiments.

B. Only enough water to quench thirst, preferably mixed with acid fruit juices.

C. In serious acute febrile conditions and during healing crises no food whatever.

D. In diseases affecting the digestive organs fasting must be prolonged several days beyond cessation of febrile symptoms.

E. Great care must be observed when breaking fast.

III. Water Treatment

A. Cooling sprays or sponge baths whenever temperature rises.

B. Fever and inflammation must not be suppressed by cold-water applications, but kept below the danger point.

C. Neither ice nor hot applications should be used.

D. Wet packs followed by cold ablutions for elimination of systemic poisons.

E. Separate compresses over seat of inflammation, also at nape of neck.

F. Kind and duration of pack to be determined by condition of patient and object to be attained.

G. Injections of tepid water to relieve constipation when necessary.

IV. Medications

A. No poisonous drugs, nor any medicines or applications which may check or suppress the feverish, inflammatory processes.

B. Homeopathic medicines, herb decoctions and specific nutritional remedies when indicated.

V. Manipulative Treatment

A. Osteopathy, massage or magnetic treatment when indicated and available.

VI. Mental Attitude

A. Courage, serenity and presence of mind are important factors.

B. Fear and anxiety intensify disease conditions, poison the secretions of the body and inhibit the action of the healing forces.

C. Do not suppress acute inflammatory and feverish processes by the power of the will.

D. The right mental and emotional attitude of relatives and friends exerts a powerful influence upon the patient.

Chapter XIV

The True Scope of Medicine

Anyone able to read the signs of the times cannot help observing the powerful influence which the Nature Cure philosophy is already exerting upon the trend of modern medical science. In Germany the younger generation of physicians has been forced by public demand to adopt the natural methods of treatment and the German government has introduced them in the medical departments of its army and navy.

In English-speaking countries, the foremost members of the medical profession are beginning to talk straight Nature Cure doctrine, to condemn the use of drugs and to endorse unqualifiedly the Nature Cure methods of treatment. In proof of this I quote from an article by Dr. William Osler in the *Encyclopedia Americana,* Vol. X, under the title of "Medicine":

Dr. Osler on Medicine

"The new school does not feel itself under obligation to give any medicines whatever, while a generation ago not only could few physicians have held their practice unless they did, but few would have thought it safe or scientific. Of course, there are still many cases where the patient or the patient's friends must be humored by administering medicine or alleged medicine where it is not really needed, and indeed often where **the buoyancy of mind which is the real curative agent,** can only be created by making him wait hopefully for the expected action of medicine; and some physicians still cannot unlearn their old training. But the change is great. **The modern treatment of disease relies very greatly on the old so-called natural methods, diet and exercise, bathing and massage**—in other words, giving the natural forces the fullest scope by easy and thorough nutrition, increased flow of blood and removal of obstructions to the excretory systems or the circulation in the tissues.

"One notable example is typhoid fever. At the outset of the nineteenth century it was treated with 'remedies' of the extremest violence—bleeding and blistering, vomiting and purging, and the administration of antimony and mercury, and plenty of other heroic remedies. Now the patient is bathed and nursed and carefully tended, but rarely given medicine. This is the result partly of the remarkable experiments of the Paris and Vienna schools in the action of drugs, which have shaken the stoutest faiths; and partly of the constant and reproachful object lesson of homeopathy. No regular physician would ever admit that the homeopathic preparations, 'infinitesimals,' could do any good as direct curative agents; and yet it was perfectly certain that homeopaths lost no more of their patients than others. **There was but one conclusion to draw— that most drugs had no effect whatever on the diseases for which they were administered."**

Dr. Osler is probably the greatest medical authority on drugs now living. He was formerly professor of materia medica at the Johns Hopkins University of Baltimore, U. S., and now holds a professorship at Oxford University, England. His books on medical practice are in use in probably every university and medical school in English-speaking countries. His views on drugs and their real value as expressed in this article should be an eye-opener to those good people who believe that we of the Nature Cure school are altogether too radical, extreme, and somewhat cranky.

However, what Dr. Osler says regarding the "New School" is true only of a few advanced members of the medical profession.

On the rank and file, the idea of drugless healing has about the same effect as a red rag on a mad bull. There are still very few physicians in general practice today who would not lose their bread and butter if they attempted to practice drugless healing on their patients. Both the profession and the public will need a good deal more education along Nature Cure lines before they will see the light.

In the second sentence of his article, **Dr. Osler admits the efficacy of mental therapeutics and therapeutic faith as a "curative agent,"** and ascribes the good effects of medicine to their stimulating influence upon the patient's mind rather than to any beneficial action of the drugs themselves.

With regard to the origin of the modern treatment of typhoid fever, however, the learned doctor is either misinformed or he misrepresents the facts. The credit for the introduction of hydropathic treatment of typhoid fever does not belong to the "remarkable experiments of the Paris and Vienna schools." These schools and the entire medical profession fought this treatment with might and main. For thirty years Priessnitz, Bilz, Ruhne, Father Kneipp and many other pioneers of Nature Cure were persecuted and prosecuted, dragged into the courts and tried on the charges of malpractice and manslaughter for using their sane and natural methods. Not until Dr. Braun of Berlin wrote an essay on the good results obtained by the hydropathic treatment of typhoid fever and it had in that way received orthodox baptism and sanction, was it adopted by advanced physicians all over the world.

Through the Nature Cure treatment of typhoid fever, the mortality of this disease has been reduced from over fifty percent under the old drug treatment to less than five percent under the water treatment.

But the average medical practitioner has not yet learned from the Nature Cure school, that **the same simple fasting and cold water which cure typhoid fever so effectively, will just as surely and easily cure every other form of acute disease,** as, for instance, scarlet fever, diphtheria, smallpox, cerebrospinal meningitis, appendicitis, etc. **Therefore, we claim that there is no necessity for the employment of poisonous drugs, serums and antitoxins for this purpose.**

Referring to the last two sentences of Dr. Osler's article, homeopaths have, as a matter of fact, lost **less** patients than allopaths. The effect of homeopathic medicine, moreover, is not altogether negative, as Dr. Osler implies. The discovery of the minute cell as the basis of the human organism on the one hand and of the unlimited divisibility of matter on the other hand explains the rationality of the infinitesimal dose. Health and disease are resident in the cell; therefore, the homeopath doctors the cell, and the size of the dose has to be apportioned to the size of the patient.

When Dr. Osler says that most drugs have no effect whatsoever, he makes a serious misstatement. While they may not contribute anything to the cure of the disease for which they are given, they are often very harmful in themselves.

Almost every virulent poison known to man is found in allopathic prescriptions. It is now positively proved by the **Diagnosis from the Eye** that these poisons have a tendency to accumulate in the system, to concentrate in certain parts and organs for which they have a special affinity and then to cause continual irritation and actual destruction of tissues. By far the greater part of all chronic diseases are created or complicated on the one hand by the suppression of acute diseases by means of drug poisons, and on the other hand through the destructive effects of the drugs themselves.

Dr. Schwenninger, the medical adviser of Prince Bismarck, and later of Richard Wagner, the great composer, has published a book entitled *The Doctor*. This work is the most scathing arraignment and condemnation of modern medical practice, especially of poisonous drugs and of surgery. Dr. Treves, the body physician of the late King Edward of England, is no less outspoken in his denunciation of drugging than Drs. Osler and Schwenninger.

Just a few men like these, foremost in the medical profession, who have achieved financial and scientific independence, can afford to speak so frankly. The great majority of physicians, even though they know better, continue in the old ruts so as to be considered ethical and orthodox, and in order to hold their practice. **It is not the medical profession that has brought about this reform in the treatment of typhoid fever and other diseases. They have been forced into the adoption of the more advanced natural methods through the pressure of the Nature Cure movement** in Germany and elsewhere.

Dr. Osler's statements, made with due deliberation in a contribution to the *Encyclopedia Americana,* are certainly a frank declaration as to the uselessness of drug treatment, and on the other hand, an unqualified endorsement of natural methods of healing.

But it seems to me that Dr. Osler pours out the baby with the bath water, as we say in German. That is, I am inclined to think that his opinion regarding the ineffectiveness of drugs is entirely too radical. **There is a legitimate scope for medicinal remedies insofar as they build up the blood on a natural basis and serve as tissue foods.**

Many people who have lost their faith in "Old School" methods of treatment have swung around to the other extreme of medical nihilism. In fact, Dr. Osler himself stands accused of being a medical nihilist.

Many of those who have adopted natural methods of living and of treating diseases have acquired an actual horror of the word medicine. However, this extreme attitude is not justified.

It also appears that some of the readers of my writings are under the impression that we of the Nature Cure school absolutely condemn the use of any and all medicines. This, however, is not so.

The Position of "Nature Cure" Regarding Medicinal Remedies

We do condemn the use of drugs insofar as they are poisonous and destructive and insofar as they suppress acute diseases or healing crises, which are Nature's cleansing and healing efforts; but on the other hand we realize that there is a wide field for the helpful application of medicinal remedies insofar as they act as foods to the tissues of the body and as neutralizers and eliminators of waste and morbid materials.

In every form of chronic disease there exists in the system, on the one hand, an excess of certain morbid materials, and on the other hand, a deficiency of certain mineral constituents, organic salts, which are essential to the normal functions of the body.

Thus, in all anemic diseases the blood is lacking in iron, which picks up the oxygen in the air cells of the lungs and carries it into the tissues, and in sodium, which combines with the carbonic acid (coalgas) that is constantly being liberated in the system and conveys it to the organs of depuration, especially the lungs and the skin. In point of fact, oxygen starvation is due in a much greater degree to the deficiency of sodium and the consequential accumulation of carbonic acid in the system (carbonic acid asphyxiation) than to the lack of iron in the blood, as assumed by the regular school of medicine.

Foods or medicinal remedies which will supply this deficiency of iron and sodium in the organism will tend to overcome the anemic conditions.

The great range of uric acid diseases, such as rheumatism, calculi, arteriosclerosis, certain forms of diabetes and albuminuria, are due, on the one hand, to the excessive use of acid-producing foods, and on the other hand, to a deficiency in the blood of certain alkaline mineral elements, especially sodium, magnesium and potassium, whose office it is to neutralize and eliminate the acids which are created and liberated in the processes of starchy and protein digestion.

In another chapter I have explained the origin and progressive development of uric-acid diseases. Our volume on Natural Dietetics will contain additional proof that practically all diseases are caused by, or complicated with, acid conditions in the system.

Any foods or medicines which will provide the system with sufficient quantities of the acid-binding, alkaline mineral salts will prove to be good medicine for all forms of acid diseases.

The mineral constituents necessary to the vital economy of the organism should, however, be supplied in the **organic** form. This will be explained more fully in subsequent pages.

From what I have said, it becomes apparent that it is impossible to draw a sharp line of distinction between foods and medicines. All foods which serve the above-named purposes are good medicines, and all nonpoisonous herb extracts, homeopathic and vitochemical remedies that have the same effect upon the system are, for the same reason, good foods.

The **medical** treatment of the Nature Cure school consists largely in the proper selection and combination of food materials. This must be so. It stands to reason that Nature has provided within the ranges of the **natural** foods all the elements which Man needs in the way of food and medicine.

But it is quite possible that, through continued abuse, the digestive apparatus has become so weak and so abnormal that it cannot function properly, that it cannot absorb and assimilate from natural foods a sufficient quantity of the elements which the organism needs. In such cases it may be very helpful and indeed imperative to take the organic mineral salts in the forms of fruit, herb and vegetable juices, extracts or decoctions. Among the best of these food remedies are extracts of leafy vegetables such as lettuce, spinach, Scotch kale, cabbage, Swiss chard, etc. These vegetables are richer than any other foods in the positive mineral salts. The extract may be prepared from one or more of these vegetables, according to the supply on hand or the tolerance of the digestive organs and the taste and preference of the patient. They should be ground to a pulp in a vegetable grinder, then pressed out in a small fruit press, which can be secured in any department store. One or two teacups per day will be sufficient to supply the needs of the system for mineral salts. This extract should be prepared fresh every day.

Then there are the Kneipp Herb Remedies. Most of these are the Hausmittel [home remedies] of the country population of Germany which have proved their efficacy since time immemorial. Their medicinal value lies in the organic mineral salts which they contain in large quantities and in beneficial combinations.

The homeopathic medications, as will be explained at length in another chapter, produce their good results because they work in harmony with the Laws of Nature.

We never hesitate, therefore, to prescribe for our patients homeopathic medicines, herb decoctions and extracts, and the vitochemical remedies which assist in the elimination of morbid matter from the system and in building up blood and lymph on a normal basis, that is, remedies which supply the organism with the mineral elements in which it is deficient in the **organic,** easily assimilable form. Herein lies the legitimate scope of medicinal remedies.

All medicinal remedies which build up the system on a normal, natural basis and increase its fighting power against disease without in any way inflicting injury upon the organism are welcome to the adherents of the Nature Cure methods of treatment.

On the other hand, we do not use any drugs or medicines which tend to hinder, check or suppress Nature's cleansing and regenerating processes. We never give anything in the least degree poisonous. We avoid all anodynes, hypnotics, sedatives, antipyretics, laxatives, cathartics, etc. Judicious fasting, cold-water applications and, if necessary, warm-water injections in case of constipation will do everything that is claimed for poisonous drugs.

Inorganic Minerals and Mineral Poisons

For many years past, physicians of the different schools of medicine, diet experts and food chemists have been divided on the question whether or not mineral substances which **in the organic form** enter into the composition of the human body may safely be used in foods and medicines in the **inorganic** form.

The medical profession holds almost unanimously that this is permissible and good practice, so that nearly every allopathic medical prescription contains some such inorganic substance, or worse than that, one or more virulent mineral poisons, as mercury, arsenic, phosphorus, etc.

So far, the discussion about the usefulness or harmfulness of inorganic minerals as foods and medicines was largely theoretical and controversial. Neither party had positive proofs for its contentions.

But Nature's records in the iris of the eye settle the question for good and for ever. One of the fundamental principles of the science of Diagnosis from the Eye is that **"nothing shows in the iris by abnormal signs or discolorations except that which is abnormal in the body or injurious to it."** When substances which are uncongenial or poisonous to the system accumulate in any part or organ of the body in sufficient quantities, they will indicate their presence by certain signs and abnormal colors in the corresponding areas of the iris.

In this way Nature makes known by her records in the eye what substances are injurious to the body, and which are harmless.

Certain mineral elements, such as iron, sodium, potassium, calcium, magnesium, phosphorus, sulphur, etc., which are among the important constituents of the human body, may be taken **in the organic form** in fruits and vegetables, or in herb extracts and the vitochemical remedies, in large amounts, in fact, far beyond the actual needs of the body, but **they will not show in the iris of the eye,** because they are easily eliminated from the system.

If, however, the same minerals be taken in the **inorganic** form in considerable quantities, the iris will exhibit certain well-defined signs and discolorations in the areas corresponding to those parts of the body in which the mineral substances have accumulated.

Obviously, Nature does not intend that these mineral elements should enter the organism in the inorganic form, and therefore the organs of depuration are not able to neutralize and eliminate them.

Thus, for instance, any amount of iron may be taken in vegetable or herb extracts, or in the vitochemical remedies, but this will not be seen in the eye. Whatever is taken in excess of the needs of the body will be promptly eliminated.

If, however, similar quantities of iron be taken for the same length of time in the inorganic, mineral form, the iron will accumulate in the tissues of stomach and bowels, and begin to show in the iris in the form of a rust brown discoloration in the corresponding areas of the digestive organs, directly around the pupil.

In similar manner sodium, which is one of the most important mineral elements in the human body, if taken in the **inorganic** form, will show in a heavy, white rim along the outer edge of the iris. Sulphur will show in the form of yellowish discolorations in the area of stomach and bowels. Iodine in the medicinal, inorganic form, prepared from the ash of seaweeds, shows in the iris in well-defined bright red spots. Phosphorus appears in whitish streaks and clouds in the areas corresponding to the organs in which it has accumulated.

An interesting exception to this rule is our common table salt (sodium chloride), which is an inorganic mineral combination. So far, diagnosticians from the eye have not discovered any sign in the iris for it. There seems to be something in its nature that makes it akin to organic substances or, like other inorganic minerals and their combinations, it would show in the iris.

This might explain why salt is the only inorganic mineral substance which is extensively used as food by humanity in general. Also animals who, guided by their natural instincts, are the finest discriminators in the selection of foods and medicines, do not hesitate to take salt freely (salt licks) when they would not touch any other inorganic mineral.

Nevertheless, we do not wish to encourage the excessive use of salt, either in the cooking of food or at the table. Taken in considerable quantities, it is undoubtedly injurious to the tissues of the body.

Before the days of canned goods, scurvy was a common disease among mariners and other people who had to subsist for long periods of time on salted meats and were deprived of fresh vegetables. The disease manifested as a breaking down of the gums and other tissues of the body, accompanied by bleeding and much soreness. As soon as these people partook of fresh fruits and vegetables, the scurvy disappeared.

The minerals contained in these organic salts foods furnished the building-stones which imparted tensile strength to the tissues and stopped the disintegration of the fleshy structures.

The Nature Cure regimen aims to provide sodium chloride as well as the other mineral elements and salts required by the body in **organic form** in foods and medicines.

When the use of inorganic minerals is discontinued and when the proper methods of eliminative treatment, dietetic and otherwise, are applied, these mineral substances are gradually dislodged and carried out of the system. Simultaneously with their elimination disappear their signs in the iris and the disease symptoms which their presence had created in the organism.

In this connection it is a significant fact that those minerals which are congenial to the system, that is, those which in their **organic** form enter into the composition of the body, are much more easily eliminated if they have been taken in the **inorganic** form, than those substances which are naturally foreign and poisonous to the human organism, such as mercury, arsenic, iodine, the bromides, the different coal-tar preparations, etc.

This is proved by the fact that the signs of the minerals which are normal constituents of the human body disappear from the iris of the eye much more quickly than the signs of those minerals which are foreign and naturally poisonous to the system.

The difficulty we experience in eliminating mineral poisons from the body would seem to indicate that Nature never intended them to be used as foods or medicines. The intestines, kidneys, skin, mucous membranes and other organs of depuration are evidently not constructed or prepared to cope with inorganic, poisonous substances and to eliminate them completely. Accordingly, these poisons show the tendency to accumulate in certain parts or organs of the body for which they have a special affinity and then to act as irritants and destructive corrodents.

The diseases which we find most difficult to cure, even by the most radical application of natural methods, are cases of drug-poisoning. Substances which are foreign to the human organism, and especially the inorganic, mineral poisons, positively destroy tissues and organs, and are much harder to eliminate from the system than the encumbrances of morbid materials and waste matter produced in the body by wrong habits of living only. The obvious reason for this is that our organs of elimination are intended and constructed to excrete only such waste products as are formed in the organism in the processes of metabolism.

Tuberculosis or cancer may be caused in a scrofulous or psoriatic constitution by overloading the system with meat, coffee, alcohol or tobacco; but as soon as these bad habits are discontinued, and the organs of elimination stimulated by natural methods, the encumbrances will be eliminated, and the much-dreaded symptoms will subside and disappear, often with surprising rapidity.

On the other hand, mercury, arsenic, quinine, strychnine, iodine, etc., accumulate in the brain, the spinal cord, and the cells and tissues of the vital organs, causing actual destruction and disintegration. The tissues thus affected are not easily rebuilt, and it is exceedingly difficult to stir up the destructive mineral poisons and to eliminate them from the system.

Therefore it is an indisputable fact that many of the most stubborn, so-called incurable diseases are drug diseases

The Importance of Natural Diet

While certain medicinal remedies in organic form may be very useful in supplying **quickly** a deficiency of mineral elements in the system, we should aim to keep our bodies in a normal, healthy condition by proper food selection and combination. A brief description of the scientific basis of "Natural Dietetics" will be found in the chapter on Diet.

Undoubtedly, Nature has supplied all the elements which the human organism needs in abundance and in the right proportions in the natural foods, otherwise she would be a very ignorant organizer and provider.

We should learn to select and combine food materials in such a manner that they supply all the needs of the body in the best possible way and thus insure perfect health and strength without the use of medicines.

Why should we attempt to cure anemia with inorganic iron, hyperacidity of the stomach with baking soda, swollen glands with iodine, the itch with sulphur, ricket conditions in infants with lime water, etc., when these mineral elements are contained in abundance and in live, organic form in fruits and vegetables, herbs and in the vitochemical remedies?

Unfortunately, however, a great many individuals, through wrong habits of living and of treating their ailments, have ruined their digestive organs to such an extent that they are incapable of properly assimilating their food and require, at least temporarily, stimulative treatment by natural methods and a supply of the indispensable organic mineral salts through medicinal food preparations.

In such cases the mineral elements must be provided in the most easily assimilable form in vegetable extracts (which should be prepared fresh every day), and in the vitochemical remedies.

What has been said is sufficient, I believe, to justify the attitude of the Nature Cure school toward medicines in general. It explains why we avoid the use of inorganic minerals and poisonous substances, while on the other hand we find a wide and useful field for medicinal remedies in the form of blood and tissue foods.

Chapter XV

Homeopathy

When we recommend the use of homeopathic remedies, the medical nihilist says: "Don't talk homeopathy to me! I didn't come to you for drugs; I have had enough of them."

When we explain that these remedies are so highly refined that they cannot possibly do any harm, he becomes still more indignant. "I don't need any of your mental therapeutics in homeopathic form," he exclaims. "I, too, believe in the power of mind over matter, but I have no faith in your sugar of milk pellets; they are poor substitutes for the real article. That kind of sugar-coated suggestion might work on some people, but it doesn't on me."

When I first entered upon the study of medicine, I, too, did not believe in the curative power of homeopathic doses; but experience caused me to change my mind. The well-selected remedy administered at the right time often works wonders.

True homeopathic medicines in high-potency doses are so highly refined and rarefied that they cannot possibly produce harmful results or suppress Nature's cleansing and healing efforts; on the contrary, if employed according to the Law of Homeopathy: "like cures like," they assist in producing acute reactions or healing crises, thus aiding Nature in the work of purification and repair.

Homeopathy Works with the Laws of Cure, Not Against Them. *Similia similibus curantur* (like cures like) translated into practice means that a drug capable of producing a certain set of disease symptoms in a healthy body, when given in large, physiological doses, will relieve or cure a similar set of symptoms in the diseased organism if the drug be given in small, homeopathic doses.

For instance, *belladonna,* given in large, poisonous doses to a healthy person, will cause a peculiar headache with sharp, stabbing pains in forehead and temples, high fever, violent delirium, dilation of the pupils, dryness and rawness of the throat, scarlet redness of the skin and extreme sensitiveness to light, jars and noises.

It will be observed that this is a fair picture of a typical case of scarlet fever. A homeopathic prescriber, when called to a scarlet fever patient exhibiting in a marked degree three or more of the above-described symptoms, would give a trituration of belladonna, say 6x. In numberless cases the fever has subsided and its symptoms have rapidly disappeared under such treatment.

The reader may say: "I do not see any difference between this and the allopathic suppression of disease by drugs."

There is a great difference. The allopathic physician may use the same remedy, belladonna, in the same case, but he will give from ten to twenty drops of tincture of belladonna, repeated every three or four hours. These doses are from twenty to forty thousand times stronger than the homeopathic 3x or 6x.

Herein lies the difference. The allopathic dose allays the fever symptoms by paralyzing the organism as a whole and the different vital organs and their functions in particular. This is frankly admitted in every allopathic materia medica. But by such dosing Nature is forcibly interrupted in her efforts of cleansing and healing; **the acute reaction is suppressed, but not cured.**

If fever is a healing effort of Nature, it may be controlled and modified, but must not be suppressed. A minute dose of homeopathic belladonna, acting on the innermost cells of the organism which the coarser allopathic doses would paralyze, stimulates these cells to effort in the right direction. It brings about conditions similar to those produced by Nature, and thus assists her; it is cooperation instead of counteroperation.

After this brief discussion of the practical application of homeopathy, let us now ascertain in how far its laws and theories agree with and corroborate the laws and principles of the Nature Cure school.

Hahnemann discovered the Law of *similia similibus curantur* accidentally, while investigating the effects of quinine on the human organism. Ever since then it has been applied successfully by him and his followers in treating human ailments.

However, this law has been used empirically. Neither in the Organon nor in any other writings or teachings of Hahnemann and the homeopathic school can be found a clear and concise explanation of why like cures like. The proof offered has been negative rather than positive.

Therefore the allopath says: "You tell me that 'like cures like,' and that you can prove it at the sickbed; but unless you can give me good and valid reasons why it should be so, I cannot and will not believe that it is your 'similar' which cures the patient. How do I know it is your 'potency'? The patient might recover just as well without it."

With the aid of the three laws of cure, I shall endeavor to give the reasons and furnish the proofs for our contentions. The laws alluded to are: **The Law of Cure, the Law of Dual Effect and the Law of Crises.**

Similia similibus curantur is only another way of stating the fundamental Law of Nature Cure: "Every acute disease is the result of a cleansing and healing effort of Nature."

If a certain set of disease symptoms are the result of a healing effort of Nature, and if I give a remedy which produces the same or similar symptoms in the system, am I not aiding Nature in her attempt to overcome the abnormal conditions?

In such a case, the indicated homeopathic remedy will not suppress the acute reaction, but it will help it along, thus accelerating and hastening the curative process.

In the last analysis, disease resides in the cell. The well-being of the organism as a whole is dependent upon the health of the individual cells of which it is composed. This has been explained more fully in connection with the action of stimulants.

In order to cure the man, we must free the cell of its encumbrances. Elimination must begin in the cell, not in the organs of depuration. Laxatives and cathartics, by irritating the digestive tract, may cause a forced evacuation of the contents of the intestinal canal, but they do not eliminate the poisons which clog cells and tissues.

In stubborn chronic diseases, when the cells are too weak to throw off the latent encumbrances of their own accord, a well-chosen homeopathic remedy is often of great service in arousing them to acute reaction.

For instance, if the system is heavily encumbered with scrofulous taints and if its vitality is lowered to such an extent that the individual cell cannot of itself throw off the morbid encumbrances by means of a vigorous, acute effort, **sulphur,** if administered in doses sufficiently triturated and refined to affect the minute cells composing the organism, will start disease vibrations similar to those of acute scrofulosis, and thus give the needed impetus to acute eliminative activity on the part of the individual cell.

The acute reaction, once started, may develop into vigorous forms of scrofulous elimination, such as skin eruptions, glandular swellings, abscesses, catarrhal discharges, etc.

Are High-Potency Doses Effective?

The question now arises: How large or how small must the dose be in order to affect the minute cells?

In the administration of medicines, the size of the dose is adjusted to the size of the patient. If half a grain of a certain drug is the normal dose for an adult, the proper dose of the same drug for a small infant, say, less than a year old, may be about one twenty-fifth of the adult dose. How small, in proportion, should then be the dose given to a cell a billion times as small as the infant?

The dose given to an adult would paralyze or perhaps kill an infant. In like manner the minute cell would be benumbed and paralyzed by the drug suited to the infant's organism.

But this is how allopathy effects its fictitious cures. It suppresses inflammatory processes by paralyzing the cells and organs and their vital activities.

Homeopathy adapts the smallness of the dose to the smallness of the cell which is to be treated. Herein lies the reasonableness of the high-potency dose.

The Personal Responsibility of the Cell

The cell resembles Man not only in physical and physiological aspects, but also in regard to the moral law.

Elimination must commence in the cell and by virtue of the cell's personal effort. Its work cannot be done vicariously by drugs or the knife. Large, allopathic doses of medicine may be given with the idea of doing the work for the cell by violently stimulating or else paralyzing the organism as a whole or certain ones of the vital organs; but this is demoralizing and destructive to the cell. The powerful doses calculated to affect the body and its organs as a whole make superfluous or paralyze the individual efforts of the cells and thus intensify the chronic disease conditions in cells and tissues.

Alms-giving, prison sentences and capital punishment have a similar allopathic effect upon Man, the individual cell of the social body. Instead of providing for him the proper environment and the opportunity for natural development and for working out his own salvation, they take this opportunity away from him and weaken his personal effort or make it impossible.

The Efficacy of Small Doses

The late revelations of chemistry, Roentgen rays, X-Rays, radioactivity of metals, etc., throw an interesting light upon the seemingly infinite divisibility of matter. A small particle of a given substance may for many years throw off a continuous shower of corpuscles without perceptibly diminishing its volume.

For an illustration we may take the odoriferous musk. A few grains of this substance will fill a room with its penetrating aroma for years. When we smell musk or any other perfume, minute particles of it bombard the end filaments of the nerves of smell in the nose. Therefore the musk must be casting off such minute particles continually without apparent loss of substance.

With the aid of this recent knowledge of the true nature of matter, of the minuteness and complexity of the atom, we can now understand how the highly triturated and refined (attenuated) homeopathic remedy may still retain the dynamic force of the element, as Hahnemann has expressed it, and how a remedy so attenuated may still be capable of exerting an influence upon the minute cell. Since chemistry and physiology have acquainted us with the finer forces of Nature, demonstrating that they are mightier than the things we can apprehend by weight and measure, the claims of homeopathy do not appear so absurd as they did a generation ago.

Undoubtedly, the good effect produced by a well-chosen remedy is heightened and strengthened by the mental and magnetic influence of the prescriber. The positive faith of the physician in the efficacy of the remedy, his sympathy and his indomitable will to assist the sufferer affect both the physical substance of the remedy and the mind of the patient.

The varying mental and magnetic qualities of prescribers have undoubtedly much to do with the varying degrees of efficaciousness of the same remedy when administered by different physicians.

The true Hahnemannian homeopath, who believes in his remedies as in his God, will concentrate his intellectual and spiritual forces on a certain remedy in order to accomplish certain well-defined results. The bottle is not allowed to become empty. Whenever the graft runs low, it is replenished with distilled water, alcohol, milk sugar, or another "vehicle." Every time he takes the medicine bottle into his hands, these potent thought forms are projected into it: "You are the element sulphur. You produce in the human body a certain set of symptoms. You will produce these symptoms in the body of this patient."

If there is any virtue at all in magnetic, mental and spiritual healing, the homeopathic remedy must be an effective agency for transmitting magnetic, mental and psychic healing forces from prescriber to patient.

Transmission of these higher and finer forces, whether directly, telepathically or by means of some physical agent, such as magnetized water, a charm or simile, etc., is the modus operandi in all the different forms of ancient and modern magic, white or black. It is the active principle in mental healing, Christian Science, sympathy healing, voodooism, witchcraft, etc.

Homeopathy and the Law of Dual Effect

I have formulated the Law of Action and Reaction in its application to the treatment of diseases as follows:

"Every agent affecting the human organism has two effects: a first, apparent, temporary one and a second, lasting one. The second effect is directly opposite to the first."

Allopathy, in giving large, physiological doses, **takes into consideration only the first, apparent effect of the drug,** and thereby accomplishes in the long run results directly opposite to those which it desires to bring about. It produces the very conditions it tries to cure. As an example, note the permanent effects of laxatives, stimulants and sedatives upon the system. This has been explained more fully in Chapter Six.

On the other hand, the homeopathic physician may use the same remedies as the allopath, provided they produce symptoms similar to those of the disease, but he administers the different drugs in such minute doses that their first effect is noticed only as a slight "homeopathic aggravation," while their second and lasting effect is relied upon to relieve and cure the disease.

In other words, **homeopathy** produces as the first effect the condition like the disease, and **counts on the second and lasting effect of the drug to bring about a permanent change.**

If, in accordance with the Law of Dual Effect as applied to drugs, the **primary,** temporary effect of the homeopathic remedy is **equal to the disease,** it is self-evident that the **secondary,** lasting effect of the remedy must be **equal to the cure.**

This law has been proved by homeopathy for over a hundred years. An experienced homeopathic prescriber would no more doubt it than he would doubt the Law of Gravitation.

Homeopathy and the Law of Crises

Therefore, if the remedy be well chosen in accord with the Law of *similia similibus curantur,* the first homeopathic aggravation, which corresponds to the crisis of Nature Cure, will be followed by speedy and perfect readjustment. Nature has her way, the disorder runs its course, and the return to normal conditions will be quicker and more perfect than if the homeopathic remedy had not been employed or if Nature's healing processes had been forcibly interrupted and suppressed by large, poisonous allopathic doses. Homeopathy assists Nature in removing the old encumbrances, whereas allopathy changes the acute, inflammatory healing effort into chronic, destructive disease.

The Economics of Homeopathy

The Law of *like cures like* is of great practical importance from another point of view, namely, that of economics.

The best engineer is the one who accomplishes the maximum of results with the minimum of expenditure of force and with the least friction. The same is true of the physician and his remedies.

We have learned that drugs given in the coarse allopathic doses attack and affect the organism as a whole. If, for instance, there is a catarrhal affection of the serous and mucous membranes of the respiratory tract accompanied by fever, the allopath will give quinine in large doses to change this condition. He may accomplish his aim; but if so, he does it by paralyzing the heart, the respiratory centers, the red and white blood corpuscles and the excreting cells of the mucous membranes. The body as a whole and certain parts in particular are saturated with the drug poison and correspondingly weakened. As allopathy itself states it: "Quinine reduces fever by depressing the metabolism" (the vital functions).

Homeopathic materia medica teaches that *Bryonia* has a special affinity for the mucous and serous membranes of the respiratory tract and that its symptomatic effects correspond closely to those described in the preceding paragraph.

If, in accordance with the Law of *similia similibus curantur,* a homeopathic dose of Bryonia be given to a patient exhibiting these symptoms, the remedy, as has been demonstrated, will assist Nature in her work of cure; and in doing this, it will not attack and affect the entire organism, but only those serous and mucous tissues for which it has a special affinity and which, as in the case of this patient, are the most seriously affected.

To state it in another way: **the large, allopathic dose paralyzes the whole organism** in order to produce its fictitious cure. **The small, homeopathic dose,** on the other hand, **goes right to the spot where it is needed,** and by mild and harmless stimulation of the affected parts, assists and supports the cells in their acute eliminative efforts.

Homeopathic medication, therefore, is not only curative in its effects, but also conservative and in the highest degree economic.

Homeopathy, a Complement of Nature Cure

Having proved the accuracy of Hahnemann's Law of *similia similibus curantur,* and having occasion daily to observe its practical results in the treatment of acute and chronic diseases, we should not be justified in omitting homeopathy from our system of treatment. The attenuated homeopathic doses of certain drugs may be of great service in bringing about the acute reactions which we so earnestly desire, especially in the treatment of chronic diseases of long standing.

I am aware of the fact that in severe and obstinate conditions homeopathy is often apparently of no avail. But when the system has been purified and strengthened by our natural methods, by a rational vegetarian diet, hydrotherapy, chiropractic or osteopathy, massage, corrective exercise, air and sun baths, normal suggestion, etc., the homeopathic remedies will work with much greater promptitude and effectiveness.

It is the combination of all the different healing factors which constitutes the perfect system of treatment.

No disease condition, whether apparently hopeless or not, can be called incurable unless all these different healing factors, properly combined and applied, have been given a thorough trial. It is no charlatanic boasting, but the simple truth, when we affirm that the different natural methods of treatment, as we of the Nature Cure school apply them, can and do cure so-called incurable diseases, such as tuberculosis, cancer, locomotor ataxy, epilepsy, eczema, neurasthenia, insanity and the worst forms of chronic dyspepsia and constipation, always providing that the patient possesses sufficient vitality to react to the treatment and that the destruction of vital parts and organs has not advanced too far.

Chapter XVI

The Diphtheria Antitoxin

In this country the antitoxin treatment for diplitheria is still in high favor, while in Germany, where it originated, many of the best medical authorities are abandoning its use on account of its **doubtful** curative results and **certain** destructive after-effects.

According to the enthusiastic advocates of this treatment among the "regular" physicians in this country, the antitoxin is a "certain cure" for diphtheria; but how is this claim borne out by actual facts?

The Health Bulletins sent regularly to every physician in the City of Chicago by the City Health Department show an average of from fifteen to twenty deaths every week from diphtheria treated with antitoxin.

I do not deny that the antitoxin treatment may have reduced somewhat the mortality percentage of this disease, allowing even for the great uncertainty of medical statistics. But we of the Nature Cure school claim and can prove **that the hydropathic treatment of diphtheria shows a much lower percentage of mortality than the antitoxin treatment.**

The crucial point to be considered in this connection is: **What are the after-effects of the different methods of treatment?**

This is a very important matter. I make the following claims:

that the antitoxin, being itself a most powerful poison, may be and often is the direct cause of paralysis, or of death due to heart-failure.

That diphtheria treated with antitoxin may be and often is followed by paralysis, heart-failure, or lifelong invalidism of some kind after the patient has apparently recovered from the disease.

That these undesirable after-effects of diphtheria do not occur when the disease is treated by natural methods, but that they are the result of the antitoxin treatment and of its suppressive effect upon. the disease.

To prove my claims, I submit the following facts: I have in my possession clippings from newspapers from different parts of the country stating that death had followed the administration of the diphtheria antitoxin for prevention or "immunization," that is, where the individual had been in good health at the time the antitoxin was given.

Several cases of this kind created quite a sensation in Germany about fifteen years ago. Dr. Robert Langerhans, superintendent of the Moabit Hospital in Berlin, a strong advocate of the antitoxin treatment and also of vaccination, had been one of a committee of three appointed by the municipal government of the German metropolis to investigate the efficiency of the diphtheria antitoxin. As a result of his findings, he had recommended its free distribution to the poor of the City of Berlin.

Not long thereafter the doctor's cook was suddenly taken ill with severe pains in the throat and sent to the hospital. It was thought to be a case of diphtheria, and the doctor, to protect his little son, one and one-half years old, against possible infection, administered an injection of antitoxin. Shortly afterward the child developed symptoms of blood-poisoning and died of heart-failure within twenty-four hours.

It is customary in Germany to insert a death-notice in one of the local newspapers and to invite the friends of the family to the funeral. In his announcement in the columns of the "Lokalanzeiger," Dr. Langerhans stated explicitly **that his little son had died after an injection of diphtheria antitoxin for immunization.**

Another similar case is that of Dr. Pistor, a prominent Berlin physician, whose little daughter contracted a slight inflammation of the throat. The child was given an injection of antitoxin, and this was followed by a severe and protracted illness.

Very significant, in this connection, are certain utterances of Dr. William Osler in his "Practice of Medicine. " He says, on page 150:

" Of the sequelae of diphtheria, paralysis is by far the most important. This can be experimentally produced in animals by the inoculation of the toxic material produced by the bacilli. [This is the active principle in the antitoxin. Author's note] The paralysis occurs in a variable proportion of the cases, ranging from 10 to 15 and even to 20 per cent. It is strictly a sequel of the disease [of the disease treated with antitoxin?—Author's note], coming on usually in the second or third week of convalescence. . . . It may follow very mild cases; **indeed, the local lesion may be so trifling that the onset of the paralysis alone calls attention to the true nature of the disease. . . .**

"The disease is a toxic neuritis, due to the absorption of the poison. . . .

"Of the local paralysis the most common is that which affects the palate. . . . Of other local forms perhaps the most common are paralysis of the eye muscles. . . . Heart symptoms are not uncommon. . . . Heart-failure and fatal syncope (death) may occur at the height of the disease or during convalescence, even as late as the sixth or seventh week after apparent recovery."

It appears to me that the mystery of these " sequelae" can easily be explained. It is certain that a mere "sore throat, " not serious enough to be diagnosed as diphtheria, cannot produce paralysis or heart-failure; but we know positively that the antitoxin can do it and does do it. The cases that Dr. Osler refers to undoubtedly received the antitoxin treatment, because it is administered on the slightest suspicion of diphtheria, nay, even to perfectly healthy persons "for purposes of immunization."

Then is it not most likely that these "mysterious after-effects" are caused rather by the highly poisonous antitoxin than by the "sore throat?"

In my own practice, I am frequently consulted by chronic patients whose troubles date back to diphtheria "cured" by antitoxin. Among these I have met with several cases of idiocy and insanity, with many cases of partial paralysis, infantile paralysis, and nervous disorders of a most serious nature, also with various other forms of chronic destructive diseases.

In the iris of the eye, the effect of the antitoxin on the system shows as a darkening of the color. In many instances, the formerly blue or light-brown iris assumes an ashy-gray or brownish-gray hue.

My secretary who is taking this dictation and who has brown eyes, tells me that her mother informed her that up to her tenth year her eyes had been of a clear blue. About that time she had several attacks of diphtheria and a severe "second" attack of scarlet fever, which were treated and "cured" under the care of an allopathic physician. She does not remember whether she was given antitoxin, but recalls that her throat was painted and her body rubbed with oil, and that she had to take a great deal of medicine. Since that time her eyes have turned brown. They show plainly the rust-brown spots of iodine in the areas of the brain, the throat, and other parts of the body.

The effect upon the iris of the eye would be very much the same whether the attacks of diphtheria had been suppressed by antitoxin or by the old-time drug treatment. A significant fact in this connection is that, since Mrs. C. is with us, following natural methods of living and under the effects of the treatments which she has been taking regularly for several months, her eyes have become much lighter and in places the original blue is visible under the brown. The nerve rings in the region of the brain, which were very marked when she came to us, have become less defined. There is a corresponding improvement in her general health, and especially in the condition of her nerves.

In regard to my claim that **undesirable after-effects do not occur under treatment by natural methods,** I wish again to call attention to the fact that for fifty years the Nature Cure physicians in Germany have proved that hydropathic treatment of diphtheria is not followed by paralysis, heart-failure, or the different forms of chronic, destructive diseases.

This has been confirmed by my own experience in the treatment of diphtheria and other serious acute ailments.

A Reply to My Critics

My discussions of the germ-theory of disease and of the vaccine, serum, and antitoxin treatment in a series of articles entitled: "Harmonies of the Physical" and published in "Life and Action" called forth a great deal of adverse criticism from physicians of the regular school of medicine. The following paragraphs are extracts from a letter sent by one of these critics to the editor of the above-named magazine:

" . . . I am convinced that some statements have been published in this particular issue [October-Decemher, 1912] which have no proper place in this magazine, the earnest champion of the cause of Truth and the official organ of expression of the U. S. headquarters of the movement which you evidently have at heart."

Dr. E. then refers to certain passages in my article in the October-December, 1912, number of "Life and Action," and comments upon them by quoting Drs. Osler and Andrews in favor of the antitoxin treatment in diphtheria and by giving his own opinion on the subject. He concludes his arguments as follows:

"I am a subscriber to this magazine and have also had my sister's name put on the mailing list. She has a little boy about two years old. Now, suppose she should read that article of Dr. Lindlahr's, and as a result, refuse to permit the use of antitoxin, and if the boy should get diphtheria, with a fatal issue as a result, I could hardly feel gratified over the fact that I had placed that reading-matter at her disposal. I fully appreciate the fact that such an unhappy result might easily ensue in some one or more of the families who read 'Life and Action' and look upon its columns as a source of the truly higher light."

Perhaps Dr. E. has not read one of Dr. Osler's latest and strongest utterances, his unqualified endorsement of natural methods of healing in the Encyclopedia Americana, quoted on page 154 of this volume.

Nature Cure in Germany

That it is possible to cure all kinds of serious acute diseases by drugless methods of healing, has been proved by the Nature Cure practitioners in Germany, nearly all of whom were laymen who had never visited a medical school. For over half a century, many thousands of them have been practicing the art of healing in all parts of Germany. With hydrotherapy and the other natural methods they have treated successfully typhoid fever. diphtheria, smallpox, appendicitis, cerebro-spinal meningitis and all other acute diseases.

It is a significant fact that, in spite of the most strenuous opposition and appeal to the law-making powers on the part of the regular school of medicine, the lay doctors could not be prevented from practicing the natural methods of treatment in law- and police-ridden Germany.

On the contrary, during the last few generations there have been practicing in Germany at all times an ever increasing number of Nature Cure physicians, most of them laymen.

This freedom of Nature Cure practice in Germany is entirely due to the success of its methods.

And this success has been demonstrated in spite of all kinds of opposition and attempted restriction. While the Nature Cure practitioner is permitted to treat those who come to him for relief, he does not have the right to cover his mistakes with six feet of earth. If one of his patients dies, a doctor of the regular school of medicine has to be called in to testify to the fact and issue the death-certificate.

Thus the "lay doctors," the "Nature Cure physicians," were and are at present constantly exposed to the strictest critical supervision by the "regulars," and if the latter can prove that a patient has died because the natural methods were inefficient or harmful, the lay practitioner can be prosecuted for and convicted of malpractice or manslaughter.

But in point of fact, while a number of these lay physicians were brought before the courts, in no instance could the actual harmfulness of the methods employed by them be proven. The natural methods of treatment became so popular that, as a matter of self-preservation, the younger generation of physicians in Germany had to fall in line with the Nature Cure idea in their practice.

Since Dr. E. so strongly questions the efficacy of our methods, I may be permitted to say something about my own professional experience.

Nature Cure in America

During the last ten years, I have treated and cured all kinds of serious acute diseases without resorting to allopathic drugs. In a very extensive practice, I have not in all these years lost a single case of appendicitis (and not one of them was operated upon), of typhoid fever, diphtheria, smallpox, scarlet fever, etc., and only one case of cerebrospinal meningitis and of lobar pneumonia. These facts may be verified from the records of the Health Department of the City of Chicago.

After the foregoing statements, I leave it to my readers to judge whether the Nature Cure philosophy is inspired by blind fanaticism and based upon ignorance and inexperience, or whether it is justified in the light of scientific facts advanced by the Regular School of Medicine itself and demonstrated by the wonderful success of the Nature Cure movement in Germany, which in its different forms has attained worldwide recognition and adoption.

There is a popular saying: "The proof of the pudding is in the eating." The following letter will explain itself:

January 20, 1913.

Dear Dr. Lindlahr:—

You may remember that last winter, Mrs. White and I attended your Sunday afternoon lectures in the Schiller Building. Those lectures were an education—I might better say a revelation and an inspiration.

On the 11th of November last, our boy, aged thirteen years, was taken ill with diphtheria. I called at your office and asked your advice. You replied: "You know what to do—wet packs, no food except fruit juices, osteopathic treatment and no antitoxin."

We called an osteopathic physician, who at once sent a specimen from the boy's throat to the city laboratory, where it was pronounced diphtheria. A physician from the Board of Health came and quarantined us and inquired if we had used the antitoxin treatment. When Mrs. White replied "No," he said: "I suppose you know that the percentage of deaths of those who do not have it is very high." She said: "Yes, I know, but we do not intend to use it."

The boy had all the acute symptoms, was drowsy, with headache, and on the second day his temperature went to 105 degrees. We applied the wet body pack and by night had reduced his temperature to 100 degrees. With the aid of the osteopathic treatment, which he had each night, the boy slept well all through big illness. On the fifth day, the membrane spread from his throat to his nose, and his temperature rose again; but the wet body packs again reduced it so that it was never again over

100 degrees.

The boy was bright, his mind was clear, he was able to read, and after the first week was able to play chess with his mother. The only unfavorable symptom he had at all was an irregular pulse. He took no medicine and no food except fruit juices. We used occasionally the warm water enema. On the tenth day he took a little lamb broth, but refused it the next day, and again asked for fruit juices. It was not until two weeks had passed that his appetite returned and he began to eat. He lost flesh, but did not lose strength in the same degree—he was able to go to the bathroom each day unaided.

On the 21st day, the osteopathic physician sent a specimen to the city laboratory which they pronounced "positive," and the city physician found it necessary to take as many as four or five additional specimens before he pronounced him free from the diphtheria germ. The boy was not released from quarantine until five weeks had passed.

During all this time his only attendant was his mother and the osteopathic physician who came daily. The boy has fully recovered and has suffered no bad results that often follow such diseases.

In contrast to this experience of ours, I would like to cite the case of a neighbor of ours whose little girl died of the disease under the antitoxin treatment. She recovered from the diphtheria, but her heart failed and she died suddenly. They had a regular M. D. and a trained nurse. Her mother took ill, but recovered. The father told me that their drug bill alone amounted to $75.

We want to express to you our gratitude for the knowledge and confidence that you have so freely given to us, and you are at liberty to make whatever use of this letter that you desire.

Sincerely yours,
HINTON WHITE
1443 Cuyler Ave., Chicago, Ill.

This letter proves that my claims and assertions regarding the curability of diphtheria by natural methods are not extravagant or untrue. In this case, as in many others, I gave directions for treatment verbally and over the telephone without having seen the patient personally.

I am convinced, furthermore, that this patient would have made just as good a recovery without the osteopathic treatment. I recommended the attendance of an osteopathic physician in order to ease the burden of responsibility on the part of the parents. If the child had died, they would have been blamed by friends and relatives for their seeming foolhardiness.

The experience of Mr. White's neighbor is another proof of the fatal effect of the antitoxin treatment. The antitoxin "cured" the diphtheria, but—the child died!

Once more I repeat: The hydropathic treatment will give equally good results in appendicitis, meningitis, scarlet fever, and all other forms of acute diseases. If this be a fact, why should not my colleagues of the Regular School of Medicine give the hydropathic method a fair trial, the more so since in Germany, even among the physicians of the Regular School, hydropathy as a remedy is fast superseding antitoxin! Is it not worth while when the "mysterious sequelae" referred to by Dr. Osler, and the many cases of chronic invalidism which he does not connect with the disease or its treatment, might thus be avoided?

Chapter XVII

Vaccination

The pernicious aftereffects of **vaccination** upon the system are similar to those of the various serum and antitoxin treatments.

Jenner, an English barber and chiropodist, is usually credited with the discovery of vaccination. The doubtful honor, however, belongs in reality to an old Circassian woman who, according to the historian Le Duc, in the year 1672 startled Constantinople with the announcement that the Virgin Mary had revealed to her an unfailing preventive against the smallpox.

Her specific was inoculation with the genuine smallpox virus. But even with her the idea was not an original one, because the principle of isopathy (curing a disease with its own disease products) was explicitly taught a hundred years before that by Paracelsus, the great genius of the Renaissance of learning of the Middle Ages. But even he was only voicing the secret teachings of ancient folklore, sympathy healing and magic dating back to the Druids and Seers of ancient Britain and Germany.

The Circassian seeress cut a cross in the flesh of people and inoculated this wound with the smallpox virus. Together with this she prescribed prayer, abstinence from meat and fasting for forty days.

As at that time smallpox was a terrible and widespread scourge, the practice of inoculation was carried all over Europe. At first the operation was performed by women and laymen; but when vaccination became popular and people were willing to pay for it, **the doctors** began to incorporate it into their regular practice.

Popular superstitions run a very similar course to epidemics. They have a period of inception, of virulence and of abatement. As germs and bacteria become inactive and die a natural death in their own poisonous excreta, so popular superstitions die as a natural result of their own falsities and exaggerations.

It soon became evident that inoculation with the virus did not prevent smallpox, but, on the contrary, frequently caused it; and therefore the practice gradually fell into disuse, only to be revived by Jenner about one hundred years later in a modified form. He substituted cowpox virus for smallpox virus.

Modern allopathy, in applying the isopathic principle, gives **large**

and poisonous doses of virus, lymph, serums and antitoxins, while homeopathy, as did ancient mysticism, applies the isopathic remedies **in highly diluted and triturated doses only.**

From England vaccination gradually spread over the civilized world and during the nineteenth century the smallpox disease (variola) constantly diminished in virulence and frequency until today it has become of comparatively rare occurrence.

"Therefore vaccination has exterminated smallpox," say the disciples of Jenner.

Is that really so? Is vaccination actually a preventive of smallpox? This seems very doubtful when the advocates of vaccination themselves do not believe it. "What," I hear them say, "we do not believe in our own theory?" Evidently you do not, my friends. If you believe that vaccination protects you against smallpox, why are you afraid of catching it from those who are not vaccinated? If you are thoroughly protected, as you claim to be, how can you catch the disease from those who are **not** protected? Why do you not allow the other fellow to have his fill of smallpox and then enjoy a good laugh on him? The fact of the matter is you know full well that **you are not safe,** that you can catch the disease just as readily as the unprotected.

German statistics are more reliable than those of any other country. In the years of 1870-71 smallpox was rampant in the Fatherland. Over 1,000,000 persons had the disease, and 120,000 died. Ninety-six percent of these had been vaccinated and only four percent had not been protected. Most of the victims were vaccinated, once at least, **shortly before they took the disease.**

In 1888 Bismarck sent an address to the governments of all the German states in which it was admitted **that numerous eczematous diseases, even those of an epidemic nature, were directly attributable to vaccination** and that the origin and cure of smallpox were still unsolved problems.

In this message to the various legislatures the great statesman said: "The hopes placed in the efficacy of the cowpox virus as a preventive of smallpox have proved entirely deceptive."

Realizing this to be a fact, most of the German governments have modified or entirely relinquished their compulsory vaccination laws.

"But," our opponents insist, "you cannot deny that smallpox has greatly diminished since the almost universal adoption of vaccination."

Certainly the disease has diminished. But so have diminished and, in fact, nearly disappeared **the plague,** the **Black Death, cholera,** the bubonic plague, yellow fever and numerous other epidemic pests which only recently decimated entire nations.

Not one of these epidemics was treated by vaccination. Why, then, did they abate and practically disappear?

Not vaccination, but the more universal adoption of soap, bathtubs, all kinds of sanitary measures, such as plumbing, drainage, ventilation and more hygienic modes of living generally have subdued smallpox as well as all other plagues.

Many of us remember how the yellow fever raged in Havanna during the Spanish occupancy. Within two months after the energetic Yankees took possession and gave the filthy city a good scouring, yellow fever had entirely disappeared—without any yellow fever vaccination.

The question is now in order why, of all the dreaded plagues of the past, smallpox alone survives to this day.

The answer is: **on account of vaccination.** If scrofulous and syphilitic poisons were not artificially kept alive in human blood by vaccination, smallpox would by this time be as rare as cholera and yellow fever.

Thanks to the oft-repeated compulsory vaccination of every citizen, young and old, we as a nation have become saturated with the smallpox virus. Is it any wonder that every once in a while this latent taint breaks out in acute epidemics?

Undoubtedly, the almost universal systematic contamination and degeneration of vital fluids and tissues, not alone with vaccine virus, but also with many other filthy serums, antitoxins and drug poisons, account in a large measure for the steady increase of tuberculosis, cancer, insanity and a multitude of other chronic destructive diseases unknown among primitive people that have not come in contact with the blessings (?) of vaccination.

By weakening the system's reactionary powers against **one** disease, its reactionary powers against all diseases are weakened. In other words, creating in the body a form of chronic smallpox by means of vaccination favors the development of all kinds of chronic diseases.

Quit sowing the seed, gentlemen, and you will cease reaping the harvest. By the mercurial suppression of syphilis and by means of vaccination **you are perpetuating smallpox**.

What has syphilis to do with smallpox? They are very closely related, and similar in appearance, symtomatology and in their effects upon the organism.

A German physician, Dr. Cruwell, who studied the subject thoroughly, says: "Every vaccination with so-called cowpox virus means syphilitic infection. Cowpox is not a disease peculiar to cattle; it is always due to syphilitic or smallpox infection from the diseased hands of human beings. Cowpox pustules have been found only on the udders of milk cows which came in contact with human hands. Cattle roaming in pasture and prairie have never been affected by cowpox, nor have domesticated steers and oxen. If this disease were a disorder peculiar to cattle, both sexes would be equally affected. Jenner's cowpox was caused by the diseased hands of the syphilitic milkmaid, Sarah Nehnes."

Vaccination of healthy children and adults is often followed by a multitude of symptoms which cannot be distinguished from syphilis, viz., characteristic ulcers and eczematous eruptions, swellings of the axillary and other lymphatic glands, atrophy of the mammary glands in the breasts of women and of girls above the age of puberty, etc.

This explains the constantly growing demand for "bust foods" and "bust developers." A perfectly developed bust has become so rare that many hundreds of beauty doctors and of business concerns that make a specialty of developing the flat-bosomed realize thousands of dollars annually. One firm in this city, and a small concern at that, has made from $2,500 to $5,000 a year and has over ten thousand names on its constantly increasing list of patrons.

It is reasonable to assume that almost without exception these ten thousand women had been vaccinated from one to three times before the age of puberty. When this is realized, and the fact that vaccination dries up the mammary glands is taken into account, is it not time to pause and consider?

The figures of this one small concern represent the report of only one out of several hundred such firms doing business in all parts of the country.

Some years ago, a disease similar to smallpox broke out among the sheep in certain parts of Scotland. As a preventive, the sheep were vaccinated. **In the course of a few years it was noticed that a great many ewes were unable to nourish their lambs.** With the discontinuance of vaccination this phenomenon disappeared.

Does this help to explain why nowadays over fifty percent of **human** mothers are incapable of nursing their babies?

Looking Forward

At present the trend of allopathic medical science is undoubtedly toward the serum, antitoxin and vaccine treatment. Practically all medical research tends that way. Every few days we see in the daily papers reports of new serums and antitoxins which are claimed to cure or create immunity to certain diseases.

Suppose the research and practice of medical science continue along these lines and are generally accepted or, as the medical associations would have it, forced upon the public by law. What would be the result? Before a child reached the years of adolescence, it would have had injected into its blood the vaccines, serums, and antitoxins of small-pox, hydrophobia, tetanus (lockjaw), cerebro-spinal meningitis, typhoid fever, diphtheria, pneumonia, scarlet fever, etc.

If allopathy were to have its way, the blood of the adult would be a mixture of dozens of filthy bacterial extracts, disease taints and destructive drug poisons. The tonsils and adenoids, the appendix vermiformis and probably a few other parts of the human anatomy would be extirpated in early youth under compulsion of the health departments.

What is more rational and sensible: the endeavor to produce immunity to disease by making the human body the breeding ground for all sorts of antibacteria and antipoisons, or to create **natural** immunity by building up the blood on a normal basis, purifying the body of morbid matter and poisons, correcting mechanical lesions and by cultivating the right mental attitude? Which one of these methods is more likely to be disease-building, which health-building?

Just imagine what human blood will be like in coming generations if this artificial contamination with all sorts of disease taints and drug poisons is to be forced upon the people!

Chapter XVIII

Surgery

The discoverers of anesthetics are classed among the greatest bene-factors of humanity, because it is believed that ether, chloroform, cocaine and similar nerve-paralyzing agents have greatly lessened the sum of human suffering. I doubt, however, that this is true.

Anesthetics have made surgery technically easy and have done away with the pain caused directly by the incisions; but on the other hand, these marvelous effects of pain-killing drugs have encouraged indiscriminate and unnecessary operations to such an extent that at least nine-tenths of all the surgical operations performed today are uncalled for. In most instances these ill-advised mutilations are followed by life-long weakness and suffering, which far outweigh the temporary pains formerly endured when unavoidable operations were performed without the use of anesthesia.

We do not wish to be understood as condemning unqualifiedly any and all surgical interventions in the treatment of human ailments. An operation may occasionally be absolutely necessary as a means of saving life. Surgery is also indicated in cases of injury, such as wounds or fractured bones, in certain obstetrical complications and in other affections of a purely mechanical nature.

In all such cases anesthetics prevent much suffering which cannot be avoided in any other way. But anyone who has had an opportunity to watch the prolonged misery of the victims of uncalled-for operations will not doubt that anesthesia has been a two-edged sword which has inflicted many more wounds than it has healed.

Many physicians have recognized more or less distinctly the use-lessness and harmfulness of "Old School" medical treatment. Dissatisfied and disgusted with old-fashioned drugging, they turn to surgery, convinced that in it they possess **an exact scientific method** of curing ailments. They seem to think that the surest way to cure a diseased organ is to remove it with the knife—fine reasoning for school boys, but not worthy of men of science.

I, for my part, cannot understand how an organ can be cured after it has been extirpated and, preserved in alcohol, adorns the specimen cabinet of the surgeon.

Destruction or Cure—Which Is Better?

"But," the surgeon says, "we do not remove organs from the body unless they have become useless."

However, this claim is not borne out by actual facts. During the past ten years thousands of patients have come under our treatment, both in the sanitarium and in the downtown offices, whose family physicians had declared that in order to save their lives they must submit to the knife without delay. With very few exceptions these people were cured by us without using a poisonous drug, an antiseptic or a knife.

Several women who, years ago, were confronted with removal of the ovaries, are today the joyful mothers of children. Many of our former patients, who were treated by "Old School" physicians for acute or chronic appendicitis and were strongly urged to have the offending organ removed, are today alive and well and still in possession of their vermiform appendices. Other patients were threatened with operations for kidney, gall and bladder stones; fibroid and other tumors; floating kidneys; stomach troubles; intestinal and uterine disorders, not to mention the multitude of children whose tonsils and adenoids were to have been removed. All of these onetime surgical cases have escaped the knife and are doing very well indeed with their bodies intact and in possession of the full quota of organs given them by Nature.

Is it not better to **cure** a diseased organ than to **remove** it? Nature Cure proves every day that the better way is at the same time the easiest way.

Thousands of men and women operated upon for some local ailment which could have been cured easily by natural methods of treatment are condemned by these inexcusable mutilations to lifelong suffering. Many, if not actually suffering pain, have been unnecessarily unsexed and in other ways incapacitated for the normal functions and natural enjoyments of life.

Cases of this kind are the most pitiable of all that come under our observation. When we learn that a major operation has been performed upon a consultant, our barometer of hope drops considerably. We know from much experience that the mutilation of the human organism has a tendency to lessen the chances of recovery; such patients are nearly always lacking in recuperative power.

A body deprived of important parts or organs is forever unbalanced. It is like a watch with a spring or a wheel taken out; it may run, but never quite right; it is hypersensitive and easily thrown out of balance by any adverse influence.

The Human Body Is a Unit

We are realizing more and more that the human body is a homogeneous and harmonious whole, and that we cannot injure one part of it without damaging other parts and often the entire organism. Cutting in the vital organs means cutting in the brain. It affects the functions of the nervous system most profoundly.

A physician in Vienna has written a very interesting book in which he shows that the inner membranes of the nose are in close relationship and sympathy with distant parts and organs of the body. He located in the nose one small area which corresponds to the lungs. By irritating this area with an electric needle he could provoke asthmatic attacks in patients subject to this disease. By anesthetizing the same area he could stop immediately severe attacks of asthma and of coughing. Another area in the nasal cavity corresponds to the genital organs. The doctor proved that by electric irritation applied to this area abortions could be produced, and that by anesthesia of the same area in the nose, uterine hemorrhages could be stopped.

These and many other facts of experience throw a wonderful light upon the unity of the human organism. The body resembles a watch. You cannot injure one part of it without affecting its entire mechanism.

The evil aftereffects of surgical operations do not always manifest at once. On the contrary, the surgical treatment is frequently followed by a period of seeming improvement. The troublesome local symptoms have been removed, and aftereffects of the mutilation have not had time to assert themselves. But sooner or later the old symptoms return in aggravated form, or a new set of complications arises. The patient is made to believe that the first operation was a perfect success and that this latest crop of difficulties has nothing to do with the former, but is something entirely new. At other times he is assured that the first operation did not go deep enough, that it failed to reach the seat of the trouble and must be done over again.

And so the work of mutilation goes merrily on. The disease poisons in the body set up one center of inflammation after another. These centers the surgeon promptly removes; but the real disease, the venereal, psoriatic or scrofulous taint, the uric or oxalic acid, the poisonous alkaloids and ptomaines affecting every cell and every drop of blood in the body, these elude the surgeon's knife and create new ulcers, abscesses, inflammations, stones, cancers, etc., as fast as the old ones are extirpated.

Those who have studied the previous chapters carefully will

readily comprehend these facts. They will know that acute and sub-acute conditions represent Nature's cleansing and healing efforts, and that local suppression by drug or knife only serves to turn Nature's corrective and purifying activities into chronic disease.

The highest art of the true physician is to preserve and to restore, not to mutilate or destroy.

Chapter XIX

Chronic Diseases

The "Old School" of medical science defines **acute diseases** as those which run a brief and more or less violent course and **chronic diseases** as those which run a protracted course and have a tendency to recur.

Nature Cure attaches a broader and more significant meaning to these terms. This will have become apparent from our discussion of the causes, the progressive development and the purpose of acute diseases in the preceding pages.

From the Nature Cure viewpoint, the chronic condition is the latent, constitutional disease encumbrance, whereas acute disease represents Nature's efforts to rectify abnormal conditions, to overcome and eliminate hereditary or acquired morbid taints and systemic poisons and to reestablish normal structure and functions.

To use an illustration: In a case of permanent or recurrent itchy psoriasis, the "Old School" physician would look upon the itchy skin eruption as the chronic disease, while we should see in the external eczema an attempt of the healing forces of Nature to remove from the system the inner, latent hereditary or acquired psora, which constitutes the real chronic disease.

It stands to reason that the exterior eruptions should not be suppressed by any means whatever, but that the only true and really effective method of treatment consists in eliminating from the organism the inner, latent psoric taint. After this is accomplished, the external "skin disease" will disappear of its own accord.

As another illustration of the radical difference in our respective points of view, let us take hemorrhoids (piles). The regular physician considers the local hemorrhoidal enlargements in themselves the chronic disease, while the Nature Cure practitioner looks upon hemorrhoids as Nature's effort to rid the system of certain morbid encumbrances and poisons which have accumulated as a result of sluggish circulation, chronic constipation, defective elimination through kidneys, lungs, and skin and from many other causes.

These constitutional abnormalities, which are the real chronic disease, have to be treated and corrected. After this has been done, the hemorrhoidal enlargements and discharges will take care of themselves.

It is, therefore, absolutely irrational, and frequently followed by the most serious consequences, to surgically remove the piles or to suppress the hemorrhoidal discharges and thereby to drive these concentrated poison extracts back into the system.

In a number of cases we have traced paralysis, insanity, tuberculosis, cancer and other forms of chronic destructive diseases to the forcible suppression of hemorrhoids.

Chronic disease, from the viewpoint of Nature Cure philosophy, means that the organism has become permeated with morbid matter and poisons to such an extent that it is no longer able to throw off these encumbrances by a vigorous, acute eliminative effort. The chronic condition, therefore, represents the slow, cold type of disease, characterized by feeble, ineffectual efforts to eliminate the latent morbid taints and impediments from the system. These efforts may take the form of open sores, skin eruptions, catarrhal discharges, chronic diarrhea, etc.

If acute diseases are treated in harmony with Nature's laws, they will leave the body in a purer, healthier condition. But if the treatment is wrong, if under the "Old School" methods fever and inflammation (Nature's methods of elimination) are checked and suppressed with poisonous drugs, serums and antitoxins or if, instead of purifying and invigorating cells and tissues, the affected parts and organs are removed with the surgeon's knife, Nature is not allowed to get rid of the disease matter, and the poisonous taints and morbid encumbrances remain in the organism.

In this way originate the worst forms of chronic diseases which now afflict civilized races.

The truth of this assertion is proved by the fact that chronic diseases we know are rare among the primitive peoples of the earth, such as the early indiginous people of Africa and Australia or the Eskimos of the arctic regions. They are not found among people who do not use drugs. All the different forms of venereal disease, chronic rheumatism, chronic indigestion, etc., are unknown in those countries whose inhabitants live in harmony with Nature. The reason is that these people have not learned to suppress Nature's acute purifying and healing efforts by poisonous drugs and surgical operations.

The Cell

Let us now study the actual condition of the cells, tissues and organs of the body in chronic disease.

We know that the human body is made up of billions of minute cells of living protoplasm. Though these cells are so small that they have to be magnified under the microscope several hundred times before we can see them, they are independent living beings which are born, grow, eat, drink, throw off waste matter, multiply, decline and die just like the large conglomerate cell which we call Man.

Each one of these little cells has its own business to attend to, whether it be assimilation, elimination, nervous activities and functions, etc.

If these little beings are well individually, the man is well. If they are starved or ailing, the entire man is similarly affected. The whole depends upon the parts. In the human body as well as in a nation or a city, the welfare of the entire community depends upon the well-being of its individual members.

If governing bodies would realize and apply these truths, and pay more attention to providing wholesome surroundings and proper conditions of living for their subjects, to an adequate supply of pure food and a normal combination of work and rest, instead of concentrating their best efforts upon restrictive and punitive measures (allopathic treatment), there would be no social problems to solve.

It is our duty to provide the most favorable conditions of living for the little cells that make up the individual human organism. If we do that, **there will be no occasion for disease.** Natural immunity will be the result.

Herein lies the vital difference between the attitude of Nature Cure and that of the allopathic school toward disease. The latter spends all its efforts in fighting the disease symptoms, while the former confines itself to creating health conditions in the habits and surroundings of the patient, from the standpoint that the disease symptoms will then take care of themselves, that they will disappear on account of nonsupport. It is the application of the injunction "Resist not Evil" to the treatment of physical disease.

Under the influence of wrong habits of living and the suppressive treatment of diseases, all forms of waste and morbid matter (the feces of the cells), together with food, drink and drug poisons accumulate in the system, affect the cells and obstruct the tiny spaces (interstices) between them. These morbid encumbrances impinge upon and clog the blood vessels, the nerve channels and the other tissues of the body. This is bound to interfere with the normal functions of the organism, and in time lead to deterioration and organic destruction.

In this connection we wish to call attention to a difference in viewpoint between the school of osteopathy and the Nature Cure school. Osteopaths and chiropractors attribute disease almost entirely to "impingement" (abnormal pressure) upon nerves and blood vessels due to dislocations and subluxations of the vertebrae of the spine and of other bony structures. **They do not take into consideration the impingement upon and obstruction of nerve channels and blood vessels all through the system caused by local or general encumbrances of the organism with waste matter, morbid products, and poisons that have accumulated in cells and tissues.**

The Life of the Cell

Every individual cell must be supplied with food and with oxygen. These it receives from the red arterial blood. The cells must also be provided with an outlet for their waste products. This is furnished by the venous circulation, which represents the drainage system of the body. If this drainage is defective, the effect upon the organism is similar to the effect produced upon a house when the excretions and discharges of its inhabitants are allowed to remain in it.

Furthermore, every cell must be in unobstructed communication with the nerve currents of the organism. Most important of all, it must be in touch with the sympathetic nervous system through which it receives the Life Force which vivifies and controls all involuntary functions of the cells and organs in the human body.

Each individual cell must be supplied with nerve fibers which convey its sensations and needs to headquarters, the nerve centers in brain and spinal cord. Also, each cell must be connected with other nerve filaments which carry impulses from the cranial, spinal and sympathetic centers to the cell, governing and directing its activities.

For instance, if the cell be hungry, thirsty, cold or in pain, it telegraphs these sensations to headquarters in the brain or spinal cord and from there directions necessary to comply with the needs of the cell are sent forth in the form of nerve impulses to the centers controlling the circulation, the food and heat supply, the means of protection, etc.

This circuit of communication from the cell over the afferent nerves to the nerve centers in the brain or spinal cord, and from these centers over the efferent nerves back to the cell or to other cells is called the reflex arc.

Let us use an illustration: Suppose the fingers come in close contact with a hot iron. The cells in the finger tips experience a sensation of burning pain. At once this sensation is telegraphed over the afferent nerves to the nerve centers in the brain or spinal cord. In response to this call of distress the command comes back over the efferent nerve filaments: "Withdraw the fingers!" At the same time the impulse to withdraw the fingers is sent over the motor nerves to the muscles and ligaments which control the movements of the hand.

If the means of communication between the different parts of the organism are obstructed or cut off entirely, the individual cell is bound to deteriorate and to die, just like a person lost in a barren wilderness and cut off from his fellowmen must perish.

In warfare it is a well-known fact that if one of the contending armies succeeds in cutting off the telegraphic communication of the other army with its headquarters, the activities of that other army are seriously handicapped. So the waste materials in the system, the disease taints, narcotic and alcoholic poisons, etc., obstruct the nerve passages, and thus interfere with the functions of the cell by cutting off its means of communication.

What has been said will serve to elucidate and emphasize the necessity of perfect cleanliness, inside as well as outside of the body. It justifies the dictum of Kuhne, the apostle of Nature Cure: "Cleanliness is Health." Anything that in any way interferes with or obstructs the circulation of vital fluids and nerve currents in the system is bound to create the abnormal conditions and functions which constitute disease.

When the morbid encumbrances and obstructions in the organism have reached the point where they seriously interfere with the nourishment, drainage and nerve supply of the cells, the latter cannot perform their activities properly, nor can they rid themselves of the impediment. They may be compared to people who are forced to live in bad, unwholesome surroundings and who cannot do their best work under these unfavorable conditions from which they cannot escape.

In this way originates chronic disease, which means that the cells have become incapable of arousing themselves to acute eliminative effort in the form of inflammatory febrile reactions.

In my lectures I sometimes liken the cell thus encumbered with morbid matter and poisons to a man buried in a mine under the debris of a cave in such a manner that it is impossible for him to free himself of the earth and timbers which are pinning him down. In such a predicament the man is unable to help himself. His fellow workers or his friends must come to his aid and remove the obstructing masses until he can assist them and free himself.

This is a good illustration of the condition of the cells of the body in chronic disease. They also have become unable to help themselves and need assistance until they can once more arouse themselves to self-help by means of an acute eliminative effort.

What can we do to help them? **We must endeavor in the first place to furnish the cells with the right nourishment.** We must abstain from everything that may be injurious to the body in food and drink, so as to relieve the cells of all unnecessary work.

Whatever one may think of vegetarianism as a continuous mode of living, a little consideration will make it plain that a rational vegetarian diet is the *sine qua non* in the cure of chronic diseases. It builds up the blood on a normal basis, excludes all food and drink poisons and thereby gives the organism an opportunity to throw off the old accumulations of waste and morbid materials.

In chronic disease, every drop of blood and every cell of the organism is affected. In order to produce a cure, the old tissues must be broken down and removed and new tissues built up. The more thorough the change in diet, the greater and more rapid will be the changes for the better in cells and tissues, especially if only pure and eliminating foods are used.

For these reasons it is advisable to omit most red-blooded meat while under the natural treatment. All animal flesh contains the morbid secretions and other waste products of the animal organism, and this means additional work for the cells already overburdened with systemic poisons.

Then we must work for elimination. Cold water applied to the surface of the body is the most powerful stimulant to the circulation. It actually pumps and pushes the blood through the system. One feels the blood rushing through the arteries and veins with greater force.

The **cold-water treatment** makes the skin more alive and active, stirs up and accelerates the circulation throughout the system and thus promotes the elimination of systemic poisons through the skin.

This stimulating effect of cold water upon the organism has been proved by counting the number of red blood corpuscles in a drop of blood before and after the application of the cold "blitzguss." They were found to have doubled in number. That does not mean that in an instant again as many red blood corpuscles had come into existence, but it does mean that before the cold "guss" one-half of them were dozing lazily in the corners. The cold water stirred them up, forced them into the circulation, made them travel and attend to business.

Another powerful means to promote elimination is **thorough, systematic massage.** The kneading, rolling, twisting and clapping actually squeezes the stagnant morbid matter and the waste products out of the tissues into the circulation, to be carried off through the venous drainage and allows the red blood with its nourishment and fresh supply of oxygen to flood the cells and organs.

Massage is also very effective as a means of regulating the blood supply in the system. In every chronic disease there is obstruction or congestion in some part of the organism, causing high blood pressure in the interior of the body and insufficient blood supply to the external parts, especially the extremities. Massage distributes the blood quickly and evenly.

Of great importance is **osteopathy.** All dislocations, luxations and subluxations of bones and ligaments should be corrected by expert manipulation. As a matter of fact, hardly a person can be found today whose spine is not abnormal in one way or another, just as there is hardly a single normal human eye [as far as iridology markings are concerned].

Manipulative treatment adjusts the lesions of the spine and other bony structures, thus removing abnormal pressure upon the nerves and blood vessels and establishing a free and abundant flow of nerve and blood currents.

Air and light baths, by stimulating the skin in a natural manner to increased activity, also contribute to the attainment of the various good results just described.

Next comes **physical exercise.** Corrective and curative movements **combined with deep breathing** promote the combustion (oxidation) of morbid materials and in this way facilitate their elimination from the system.

Life itself is dependent upon breathing. The Life Force enters the body with every breath we draw. Show me a man with well-developed, full-breathing lungs, and I will show you a man with good vitality.

Last but not least among the natural methods of treating the cell in chronic disease we mention **the right mental and emotional attitude.** Fear, anxiety and all kindred emotions congeal the nerve matter and thereby shut off the supply of nerve force. The cells and tissues starve and freeze. On the other hand, the emotions of hope, confidence and cheerfulness relax and open blood vessels and nerve channels and allow the free and unobstructed inflow and circulation of vital energy.

The different methods of natural treatment and their practical application in chronic diseases will be discussed in detail in subsequent chapters.

When through natural methods of living and of treatment the morbid encumbrances have been removed sufficiently to provide and maintain normal blood supply, better venous drainage and the unobstructed flow of the nerve currents, when lesions of the bony structures have been corrected by skilful adjustment, and when, through right mental attitude, a free and abundant inflow of Life Force has been established, then the cells and tissues of the body become once again able to arouse themselves to an acute eliminative effort, and the organism is ready for a healing crisis.

Chapter XX

Crises

Crisis in the ordinary sense of the word means change, either for better or for worse. In its relation to medicine, the term "crisis" has been defined as "a decisive change in the disease, resulting either in recovery or in death."

We of the Nature Cure school distinguish between healing crises and disease crises, according to the character and the tendency of the acute reaction. If an acute disease is brought about through the accumulation of morbid matter or the invasion of disease germs to such an extent that the health or the life of the organism is endangered, in other words, if the disease conditions are forcing the crises, we speak of disease crises.

But if acute reactions take place in the system because conditions have become more normal, because the healing forces have gained the ascendancy and forced the acute inflammatory processes, we call them healing crises.

Healing crises are simply different forms of elimination by means of which Nature endeavors to remove the latent, chronic disease encumbrance from the system. The most common forms of these acute purifications are colds, catarrhal and hemorrhoidal discharges, boils, ulcers, abscesses, open sores, skin eruptions, diarrheas, etc.

Healing crises and disease crises may seem very much alike. Patients often tell me: "I have had this before. I call it an ordinary boil (or cold, or fever)."

That may be true. The former disease crisis and the present healing crisis may be similar in their outward manifestations. **But they are taking place under entirely different conditions.**

When the organism is loaded to the danger point with morbid matter, it may arouse itself in self-defense to an acute eliminative effort in the shape of cold, catarrh, fever, inflammation, skin eruption, etc. In these instances, the disease conditions bring about the crisis and the organism is on the defensive. These are disease crises.

Such unequal struggles between the healing forces and disease conditions sometimes end favorably and sometimes unfavorably.

On the other hand, healing crises develop because the healing forces are in the ascendancy and take the offensive. They are brought about through the natural methods of living and of treatment and always result in improved conditions.

A simple allegory may assist me in explaining the difference between a healing crisis and a disease crisis:

For years a prizefighter holds the championship because he keeps himself in perfect physical condition and before every contest spends many weeks in careful training. When he faces his opponent in the ring, he has eliminated from his organism as much waste matter and superfluous flesh and fat as possible by a strictly regulated diet and a great deal of hard exercise. As a consequence, he comes off victorious in every contest and easily maintains his superiority.

These victories in his career, like healing crises in the organism, are the result of training and preparation.

The prizefighter in the one case and Vital Force in the other are on the offensive from the beginning of the struggle and have the best of the fight from start to finish.

Rendered overconfident by long-continued success, our champion gradually permits himself to drift into a weakened physical condition. He omits his regular training and indulges in all kinds of dissipation.

One day, full of self-conceit and underestimating the strength of his challenger, he enters the ring without preparation and is ingloriously defeated by a man who, under different circumstances, would not be a match for him.

So, in the case of a patient in a disease crisis, fatal termination may be due to the excessive accumulation of waste and morbid matter in the system, to lowered vitality and to lack of preparation. Victory or defeat in acute reactions as well as in the ring depends on right living and preparatory training.

In the healing crisis, vitality is the stronger and gains the victory in the struggle; in the disease crisis, disease conditions have gained the ascendancy and may bring about the defeat of the healing forces.

Under conditions favorable to human life, a body of normal structure, healthy blood and tissues and good vitality cannot be affected by acute disease. Such an organism is practically immune to all forms of inflammatory febrile reactions. These always indicate that there is something wrong in the system which Nature is trying to correct or get rid of.

Healing Crises

In Chapter Two "Catechism of Nature Cure," we defined "healing crises" as follows: "A healing crisis is an acute reaction, resulting from the ascendancy of Nature's healing forces over disease conditions. Its tendency is toward recovery, and it is, therefore, in conformity with Nature's constructive principle." The possibility of producing healing crises and thereby curing chronic ailments depends upon the following conditions:

1. The patient must possess sufficient vital energy and powers of reaction to respond to the natural treatment and to a change of habits.
2. The destruction and disorganization of vital fluids and organs must not have advanced too far.

Some patients become frightened at the idea of crises. They exclaim: "I came here to get well, not to grow worse."

However, there is no occasion for alarm. Healing crises occur in mild form only because, under the influence of natural living and treatment, Nature has the best of the fight. The healing forces of the organism have gained the ascendancy over the disease conditions.

In fact, **Nature never undertakes a healing crisis until the system has been prepared for it,** until the organism is sufficiently purified and strengthened to conduct the acute reaction to a favorable termination.

Furthermore, it is well to remember that crises cannot be avoided, because it is through fevers and inflammatory processes that Nature effects the cure—that she tears down the old to build up the new.

On the other hand, if patients are possessed of exceptionally good vitality and if the organs of elimination are in good working order, the purification and adjustment of the organism may occasionally proceed gradually without the occurrence of marked acute reactions or crises.

Healing Crises, When Properly Conducted, Are Never Fatal to Life

When well assisted by the right, natural methods of living and of treatment, healing crises are never dangerous or fatal to life. The only danger lies in suppressing these acute reactions by drugs, knife, the ice bag or any means whatever.

If acute reactions are suppressed, the constructive healing crisis may be changed into a destructive disease crisis. Therefore we earnestly warn our patients never to interfere in any way with a healing crisis lest the chronic condition (which resulted from the suppression of the original disease) become worse than before.

When Nature, with all the force inherent in the human organism, has finally worked up to the point of a healing crisis, another defeat by a new suppression may be beyond her powers of endurance and recuperation. Fatal collapse may then be the result.

Therefore, take heed! If you are not willing to endure the healing crises, do not undertake the treatment. When you have conjured up the hidden demons of disease, you must have the courage to face and subdue them. Nothing good in life comes to us except as we pay the price. He who is too cowardly to conquer in a healing crisis may perish in a disease crisis.

Drugs Versus Healing Crises

Our explanations of the natural laws of cure and of natural therapeutics are often greeted by "Old School" physicians and students with remarks like the following:

"You speak as if you had the monopoly of eliminative treatment and of the production of crises. With our laxatives, cathartics, diuretics, diaphoretics and tonics, we are doing the same thing. What is more effectual for stimulating a sluggish liver and cleansing the intestinal tract than calomel followed by a dose of salts? What will produce more profuse perspiration than pilocarpin; or what is a better stimulus to the kidneys than squills or buchu? Can we not by means of stimulants and depressants regulate heart action to a nicety?

"We accomplish all this in a clean, scientific manner, without resorting to unpleasant dieting and to barbarous applications of douches, packs and manual treatments. Isn't it more dignified and professional to write a Latin prescription? How much better the impression on the laity than soaking and rubbing!"

Let us see if these statements are true, if laxation, urination or perspiration produced by poisonous drugs are identical in character and in effect with the elimination produced by natural living and natural methods of treatment through healing crises.

Mercury, in the form of calomel, is one of the best-known cholagogues [an agent designed to increase the flow of bile and, thereby, stimulate lower bowel action, *ed*.]. It is the favorite laxative and cathartic of allopathy. The prevailing idea is that calomel acts on the liver and the intestines; but **in reality these organs act on the drug.**

All laxatives and cathartics are poisons; if it were not so, they would not produce their peculiar, drastic effects. Because they are poisons, Nature tries to eliminate them from the system as quickly and as thoroughly as possible. In order to do this, the excretory glands and membranes of the liver and the digestive tract greatly increase the amount of their secretions and thereby produce a forced evacuation of the intestinal canal.

Thus the system, in the effort to eliminate the mercurial poison, expels also the other contents of the intestines. This may effect a temporary cleansing of the intestinal tract, but it does not and cannot cleanse the individual cells throughout the body of their impurities.

The Lasting Effects of Artificial Purging

In accordance with the Law of Action and Reaction, action and reaction are equal and opposite; the temporary irritation and overstimulation of the sensitive membranes of the digestive organs are followed by corresponding weakness and exhaustion, and if this procedure be repeated and become habitual, by gradual atrophy and paralysis. As atrophy progresses, the dose of the purgative must be increased in order to accomplish the desired result and this, in its turn, hastens the degenerative changes in the system.

Such enforced, artificial purging may flush the drains and sewers, but does not cleanse the chambers of the house. The cells in the interior tissues remain encumbered with morbid matter. A genuine and truly effective housecleaning must start in the cells and must be brought about through the initiative of the vital energies in the organism, through healing crises, and not through stimulation by means of poisonous irritants.

When, under a natural regimen of living and of treatment, the system has been sufficiently purified, adjusted and vivified, the cells themselves begin the work of elimination.

This is what takes place: The morbid matter and poisons thrown off by the cells and tissues are carried by means of the venous circulation to the organs of elimination, the bowels, kidneys, lungs and skin, and to the mucous membranes lining the interior tracts, such as the nasal passages, the throat and bronchi, the digestive and genitourinary canals, etc.

These organs of elimination become overcrowded with the rush of morbid matter and the accompanying congestion and irritation cause the acute inflammatory processes and feverish symptoms characterizing the various forms of colds, catarrhs, skin eruptions, diarrheas, boils and other acute forms of elimination, which we call healing crises. In other words, **what the "Old School" of medicine calls the disease, we look upon as the Cure.**

Acute elimination brought about in this manner is Nature's method of housecleaning. It is a true healing crisis, **the result of purification and increased activity from within the cell, produced by natural means.**

Here interposes Friend Allopath: "You claim that you bring about your acute reactions by natural means only, and that these are never injurious to the organism. What difference does it make if the circulation is stimulated and elimination increased by a cold-water spray or by digitalis? The cold-water stimulation produces a reaction just as digitalis does, and the one must therefore be as injurious as the other."

To this we reply: "The stimulating effect on heart and circulation produced by digitalis is the first action of a highly poisonous drug; the second lasting effect is weakening and paralyzing. On the other hand, the first action of a cold-water spray is depressing; it sends the blood into the interior of the body and benumbs the surface. The sensory nerves at once report this sensation of cold to headquarters in the brain, and immediately the command is telegraphed to the blood vessels in the interior of the body: 'Send blood to the surface!' As a result, the blood is carried to the surface, and the skin becomes warm and rosy with the glow of life. In this case the stimulation is the second and lasting effect of the water treatment, from which there is no further reaction."

Similarly, the stimulation produced by exercise, massage, manipulation or the exposure of the nude body to light and air is natural stimulation, produced by harmless, natural means. It is entirely due to the fact that conditions in the system have been made more normal, as explained in other chapters.

Drugs, stimulants and tonics, while they produce an artificial, temporary stimulation, do not change the underlying abnormal conditions in the organism. Likewise, the flushing of the colon with water, the use of laxative herb teas and decoctions or forced sweating by means of Turkish or Russian baths, though not as dangerous as inorganic minerals and poisonous drugs, cannot be classed among the natural means of cure. These agents, which by many persons are looked upon as natural treatment, irritate the organs of elimination to forced, abnormal activity without at the same time arousing the cells in the interior of the body to natural elimination.

Dr. H. Lahmann, one of the foremost scientists of the Nature Cure movement, made a series of interesting experiments. His chemists gathered the natural perspiration of certain patients, produced by ordinary exercise in the sunshine. These excretions of the skin were evaporated and analyzed, and were found to contain poisons powerful enough to kill rabbits.

If profuse sweating was produced in the same patients by the high temperature of the hot-air box or the electric-light cabinet, their perspiration, when evaporated and analyzed, was found to contain only small amounts of toxins. Thus Dr. Lahmann proved that:

1. Sweating and the elimination of disease matter are two different processes.

2. Artificially induced sweating does not eliminate disease matter.

3. The organism cannot be forced by irritants and stimulants and artificial means, but eliminates morbid matter only in its own natural manner and when it is in proper condition to do so.

In a lesser degree, this applies also to fasting. Under certain conditions it becomes a necessity; but it may easily be abused and overdone.

Do We Never Fail?

Certainly we fail, but our failures are usually due to the fact that sick people, as a rule, do not consider Nature Cure except as a last resort. The methods and requirements of Nature Cure appear at first so unusual and exacting that people seek to evade them so long as they have the least faith in the miracle-working power of the poison bottle, a metaphysical healer or the surgeon's knife. When health, wealth and hope are entirely exhausted, then the chronic sufferer grasps at Nature Cure as a drowning man clutches at a straw. But even though ninety percent of these cases which come to us are of the apparently incurable type, our total failures are few and far between.

If there is sufficient vitality in the body to react to natural treatment and if the destruction of vital parts and organs has not too far advanced, a cure is possible. Often the seemingly hopeless cases yield the most readily.

Our success is due to the fact that we do not rely on any one method of treatment, but combine in our work everything that is good in the different systems of natural healing.

The Law of Crises

Everywhere in nature and in the world of men we find the Law of Crises in evidence. This proves it to be a universal law, ruling all cosmic relations and activities.

Wars and revolutions are the healing crises in the life of nations. Heresies and reformations are the crises of religion. In strikes, riots and panics, we recognize the crises of commercial life.

Staid old Mother Earth herself has in the hoary past repeatedly changed the configurations of her continents and oceans by great cataclysms or geological crises.

When the sultry summer air has become pregnant with poisonous vapors and miasmas, atmospheric crises, such as rainstorms, thunder, lightning and electric storms, cool and purify the air and charge it anew with life-giving ozone. In like manner will healing crises purify the disease-laden bodies of men.

Emanuel Swedenborg gives us a wonderful description of the Law of Crises in its relationship to the regeneration of the soul. We quote from the chapter in which he describes the working of this law, entitled, "Regeneration Is Effected by Combats in Temptation."

"They who have not been instructed concerning the regeneration of man think that man can be regenerated without temptation. But it is to be known that no one is regenerated without temptation; and that many temptations succeed, one after another. The reason is that regeneration is effected for an end, in order that the life of the old man may die, and the new life which is heavenly be insinuated. It is evident, therefore, that there must be a conflict [healing crisis—*author's note*]; for the life of the old man resists and determines not to be extinguished; and the life of the new man can only enter where the life of the old is extinct.

"Whoever thinks from an enlightened rationale, may see and perceive from this that a man cannot be regenerated without combat, that is, without spiritual temptations; and further, that he is not regenerated by one temptation, but by many. For there are very many kinds of evil which formed the delight of his former life, that is, of the old life. These evils cannot all be subdued at once and together; for they cleave tenaciously, since they have been inrooted in the parents for many ages back [the scrofula of the soul—*author's note*] and are therefore innate in man, and are confirmed by actual evils from himself from infancy. All these evils are diametrically opposite to the celestial good [perfect health—*author's note*] that is to be insinuated and which is to constitute the New Life."

Thus the inspired Seer of the North draws a vivid picture of what we call healing crises in their relation to moral regeneration.

We cannot help recognizing the close agreement of physical and spiritual crises; this, again, demonstrates the continuity and exact correspondence of Natural Law on the different planes of being. [The Law of Hermes: *As above, so below; as in the inner, so in the outer; as in the lesser, so in the greater.*]

We of the Nature Cure school know that this great Law of Crises dominates the cure of chronic disease. Every case is another verification of it; in fact, every decided advance on the road to perfect health is marked by acute reactions.

The cure invariably proceeds through the darkness and chaos of the crises to the light and beauty of perfect health, periods of marked improvement alternating with acute eliminating activity (the "spiritual temptations" and "combats" of Swedenborg), until perfect regeneration has taken place.

Chapter XXI

Periodicity

In many forms of acute disease, crises develop with marked regularity and in well-defined periodicity. This phenomenon has been observed and described by many physicians.

It is not so well known, however, that in the cure of chronic diseases also, crises develop in accordance with certain laws of periodicity.

Periodicity is governed by the Septimal Law or Law of Sevens, which seems to be the basic law governing the vibratory activities of the planetary universe.

The harmonics of heat, light, sound, electricity, magnetism and of atomic structure and arrangement run in scales of seven.

The Law of Sevens governs the days of the week, the phases of the moon and the menstrual periods of the woman. Every observing physician is aware of its influence on feverish, nervous and psychic diseases.

The Law of Sevens dominates the life of individuals and of nations and of everything that lives and has periods of birth, growth, fruitage and decline.

Over two thousand years ago Pythagoras and Hippocrates distinctly recognized and proclaimed the Law of Crises in its bearing on the cure of chronic diseases. They taught that alternating, well-defined periods of improvement and of crises were determined and governed by the law of periodicity and by the law of numbers (the Septimal Law).

The following quotations are taken from the *Encyclopedia Britannica,* Vol. XV, p. 800:

> "But this artistic completeness was closely connected with 'the third cardinal virtue' of Hippocratic medicine—the clear recognition of disease as being equally with life a process governed by what we should now call natural laws, which could be known by observation and which indicated the spontaneous and normal direction of recovery, by following which alone could the physician succeed.
>
> "Another Hippocratic doctrine, the influence of which is not even yet exhausted, is that of the healing power of Nature. Not that Hippocrates taught, as he was afterwards reproached with teaching, that Nature is sufficient for the cure of diseases; for he

held strongly the efficacy of art. But he recognized, at least in acute diseases, a natural process which the humours went through—being first of all crude, then passing through coction or digestion, and finally being expelled by resolution or crisis through one of the natural channels of the body. The duty of the physician was to foresee these changes, 'to assist or not to hinder them,' so that 'the sick man might conquer the disease with the help of the physician.' The times at which crises were to be expected were naturally looked for with anxiety; and it was a cardinal point in the Hippocratic system to foretell them with precision. Hippocrates, influenced as is thought by the Pythagorean doctrine of numbers, taught that they were to be expected on days fixed by certain numerical rules, in some cases on odd, in others on even numbers—the celebrated doctrine of 'critical days.' It follows from what has been said that prognosis, or the art of foretelling the course and event of the disease, was a strong point with the Hippocratic physicians.[2] In this perhaps they have never been excelled. Diagnosis, or recognition of the disease, must have been necessarily imperfect, when no scientific nosology, or system of disease existed, and the knowledge of anatomy was quite inadequate to allow of a precise determination of the seat of disease; but symptoms were no doubt observed and interpreted skilfully. The pulse is not spoken of in any of the works now attributed to Hippocrates himself, though it is mentioned in other works of the collection.

"In the treatment of disease, the Hippocratic school attached great importance to diet, the variations necessary in different diseases being minutely defined. . . . In chronic cases diet, exercises and natural methods were chiefly relied upon."

These wonderful truths, with other wisdom of the ancients, were lost in the spiritual darkness of the Middle Ages. Modern medicine looks upon these claims and teachings of the Hippocratic School as "superstition without any foundation in fact." However, the great sages of antiquity, drawing upon a source of ancient wisdom, deeply hidden

---

2 The author of this article in the Encyclopedia Britannica does not see that it is the modern [then as now] orthodox "scientific nosology, or system of disease" which obscures the simplicity and precision of the Hippocratic philosophy of disease and cure.

from the self-satisfied scribes and wise men of the schools, after all, proclaimed the truth.

Every case of chronic disease properly treated by **natural** methods proves the reality and stability of the Law of Crises. It is therefore a standing wonder and surprise to one who knows, that this all-important and self-evident law is practically unknown to the disciples of the regular schools.

The Law of Sevens

In accordance with the Law of Periodicity, the sixth period in any seven periods is marked by reactions, changes, revolutions or crises. It is, therefore, looked upon by popular intuition as an unlucky period. Friday, the sixth day of the week, is regarded as an unlucky day; Friday is hangman's day; according to tradition the Master, Jesus, was crucified on Friday.

Counting from the first sixth or Friday period in any given number of hours, days, weeks, months, years or groups of years, as the case may be, every succeeding seventh period is characterized by crises.

This explains why 13 is considered an unlucky number. It represents the second critical or Friday period.

However, there is really no cause for this superstitious fear of Friday and the number 13. It is due to a lack of understanding of Nature's Laws. By intelligent cooperation with these laws we may turn the critical periods in our lives into healing crises and beneficial changes.

We should not fear the crises periods of the larger life and the changes in our outward circumstances which they may bring any more than we should fear crises in the physical body.

A thorough understanding of the nature and purpose of healing crises in acute and chronic diseases has taught me the nature and purpose of evil in general. It has made me understand more clearly the meaning of "Resist not Evil" and of the saying: "We are punished **by** our sins, not **for** our sins." It has shown me that evil is not a punishment or a curse, but a necessary complement of good, that it is corrective and educational in its purposes, that it remains with us only as long as we need its salutary lessons.

The evil of physical disease is not due to accident or to the arbitrary rulings of a capricious Providence, nor is it always "error of mortal mind." From the Nature Cure philosophy and its practical applications we have learned that, barring accidents and conditions or surroundings unfavorable to human life, it is caused in every instance by violations of the physical laws of our being. So the social, political and industrial evil of the larger life is brought about by violations of the law in the respective domains of life and action.

So long as transgressions of the physical laws of our being result in hereditary and acquired disease encumbrances, we must expect reactions which may become either disease crises or healing crises. Likewise, so long as ignorance, selfishness and self-indulgence continue to create evil in other domains of life, we must expect there also the occurrence of crises, of reaction and revolution. When knowledge, self-control and altruism become the sole motives of action, evil and the crises it necessitates will naturally disappear.

Therefore, **we should not be afraid of changes and crises periods but cooperate with them clear-eyed and strong-willed.** Then they will result in improvement and further growth.

Life is growth, and growth is change. The only death is stagnation. The loss of friends, home or fortune may seem for the time being an overwhelming calamity; but if met in the right spirit, such losses will prove stepping-stones to greater opportunity and higher achievement.

Many of our patients formerly looked upon their diseased condition as a great misfortune and an undeserved punishment; but since it brought them in contact with the Nature Cure philosophy and showed them the necessity of complying with the laws of their being, they now look upon the former evil as the greatest blessing in their lives, because it taught them how to become the masters of fate instead of remaining the plaything of Nature's destructive forces.

Why should we fear even the greatest of all crises, physical death, when it, also, is only the gateway to a larger life, greater opportunities and more beautiful surroundings? Why should we mourn and grieve over the death of friends and relatives, when they have only emigrated to another, better country?

Suppose we ourselves had to enter upon the great journey today or tomorrow, shouldn't we be glad to meet some of our friends on the other side and to be welcomed, advised and guided by them in the new surroundings?

Therefore we should not fear, nor endeavor to avoid the crises in any and all domains of life and action, but meet them and cooperate with them fearlessly and intelligently. They then will always make for greater opportunity and higher accomplishment.

The Law of Sevens Applied to Individual Life

Applied to the life of the individual, the Law of Periodicity manifests itself as follows:

Human life on the earth plane is divided into periods of seven years. The first seven years represent the period of infancy. With the next seven, the years of childhood, begins individual responsibility, the conscious discernment between right and wrong. The third group comprises the years of adolescence; the fourth marks the attainment of full growth. Nearly all civilized countries take cognizance of this fact by fixing the legal age at twenty-one.

The twenty-eighth year, the beginning of the fifth period, is another milestone along the road to development.

The sixth period, beginning at the age of thirty-five and ending at forty-two, is marked by reactions, changes and crises. It may, therefore, seem an unlucky period; but if we understand the law and comply with it, we shall be better and stronger in every way after we have passed this period.

During the seventh period, the effects of the sixth or crises period continue and adjust themselves. It is a period of reconstruction, of recuperation and rest, and thus the best preparation for a new cycle of sevens which begins with the fiftieth year.[3]

In this connection it is interesting to note that the Mosaic law recognized the law of periodicity and fixed upon **Sunday as the first day or "birthday"** of the week, and upon **Saturday** (the Sabbath) **as the last or "rest" day,** in which to prepare for another period of seven days.

Orthodox science now admits that the normal length of human life should be about one hundred and fifty years. This would constitute three cycles of forty-nine years each, the first corresponding to youth, the second to maturity, and the third to fruition.

The Law of Sevens in Febrile Diseases

If we apply the Laws of Periodicity to the course of acute febrile or

3 Those who are interested in the Law of Periodicity as applied to life in general, will find much valuable information in a book entitled *Periodicity* by J. R. Buchanan, M.D., published by the Kosmos Publishing Co., 2112 Sherman Ave., Evanston, Il.

inflammatory diseases, we find that the sixth day from the beginning of the first well-defined symptom marks the first Friday-period or the first crisis of the disease, and that every seventh day thereafter is also distinguished by aggravations and changes, either for better or for worse.

The Law of Sevens in Chronic Diseases

Applied to the cure of chronic diseases under the influence of natural methods of living and of treatment, the Laws of Crises and of Periodicity manifest as follows:

When a chronic patient, whose chances of cure are good, is placed under proper (natural) conditions of living and of treatment he will, as a rule, experience five weeks of marked improvement.

The sixth week, if conditions are favorable, usually marks the beginning of acute reactions or healing crises. This means that the healing forces of the organism have grown strong enough to begin the work of acute elimination.

By all sorts of acute reactions, such as skin eruptions, diarrheas, feverish, inflammatory and catarrhal conditions, boils, abscesses, mucopurulent discharges, etc., Nature now endeavors to remove the latent, chronic disease taints from the system.

The character of the healing crises and the time of their occurrence in any given case can often be accurately predicted by means of the **Diagnosis from the Eye** (see Chapter XIII), from Nature's records in the iris.

But **the best of all methods of diagnosis is the cure iself,** because weak spots and morbid taints in the organism are revealed through the healing crises.

The Same Old Aches and Pains

Frequently we hear from a patient in the throes of crises: "These are the same old aches and pains that I had before. It is exactly the same trouble I have been suffering with for many years. This is not a crisis !—I have caught a cold, or I have eaten something which does not agree with me."

The patient has forgotten what we taught him regarding the Law of Crises. He loses sight of the fact that healing crises are nothing more or less than a coming-up-again of old disease conditions, **an acute manifestation of ailments which had become chronic through neglect or suppression.**

Of course they are "the same old aches and pains." Nature Cure does not create new diseases. Crises mean the stirring up and eliminating of hereditary and acquired taints and poisons. Under the right methods of treatment, any previous disease condition suppressed by drugs or knife or by mental effort may recur as a healing crisis.

They are the same old aches and pains which so often gave trouble in the past, **but they are now running their course under different conditions** because the patient is now living in harmony with Nature's Laws.

Under the natural regimen, Nature is encouraged and assisted in her cleansing and healing efforts. She is allowed in her own wise way to tear down the old and build up the new.

The "Old Schools" of healing proclaim Mother Nature a poor healer. But we of the Nature Cure school believe that the wisdom which created this wonderful, complex mechanism which we call the human body knows also how to preserve and to repair it. Every healing crisis passed under natural conditions assisted by natural methods of treatment leaves the body purified and strengthened and nearer to perfect health.

Our critics and opponents frequently ask us how we know that our methods are natural and in harmony with Nature's laws.

To this we reply: The timely appearance of healing crises, their orderly development and favorable termination constitute the best criterion of the correctness and naturalness of the methods of treatment employed. The prompt arrival and beneficial results of acute reactions are a certain indication that the healing forces of the organism are in the ascendancy and that the treatment is in conformity with the natural laws of cure and with the **constructive** principle in Nature.

Another question sometimes asked of us is: "Do healing crises develop in every chronic disease under natural treatment?" Our answer is: If the condition of the patient is not favorable to a cure, that is, if the vitality is too low and the destruction of vital parts too far advanced, the healing crises may be proportionately delayed or may not occur at all. In such cases the disease symptoms will increase in severity and complexity and become more destructive instead of more constructive, until the final fatal crisis. The end may come quickly, or the patient may decline gradually toward the fatal termination.

Again, patients ask us: "Through how many crises shall I have to pass?" We tell them: Just as many as you need; no more, no less. So long as there is anything wrong in the system, crises will come and go; but each crisis, if successfully passed, is another milestone on the road to perfect health.

It is intensely interesting to observe how orderly and intelligently Nature proceeds in her work of healing and repair. One problem after another is taken up and adjusted.

First of all, the digestive organs are put into better condition, because further progress depends upon proper assimilation and elimination. The bowels must act freely and naturally before any permanent improvement can take place. A treatment which fails to accomplish this first preliminary improvement will surely fail to produce more important results.

In this connection it is a significant fact that nearly all our patients, when they come under our care, are suffering from very stubborn constipation in spite of (or possibly on account of) lifelong drugging. Neither medicines nor operations had given them anything but temporary relief and the trouble had grown worse instead of better.

If the "Old School" methods of treatment were not successful in relieving simple constipation, what else can they be expected to cure, since the overcoming of constipation is evidently the primary necessity for any other improvement?

A system of treatment which cannot accomplish this cannot accomplish anything else. It is strange, therefore, that a school of medicine which has not succeeded, with all its vaunted knowledge and wisdom, to cure simple constipation, flatly denies that natural methods can cure cancer, epilepsy, locomotor ataxy and other so-called incurable diseases.

Our Greatest Difficulty

The greatest difficulty in our work lies in conducting our patients safely through the stormy crises periods. The first, preliminary improvement is often so marked that the patient believes himself already cured. He will say: "Doctor, I am feeling fine! There is nothing the matter with me any more! I cannot understand why I shouldn't go home and continue the natural regimen there!"

This feeling of mental elation and physical well-being is usually the sign that the first general improvement has progressed far enough to prepare the system for a healing crisis. Therefore my answer to the overconfident patient may be something like this: "Remember what I told you. The first improvement is not the cure, it is only the preparation for the real fight. Look out! In a few days you may whistle another tune."

And sure enough, usually within a few days after such a conversation the patient is down in the slough of despond. His digestive organs are in a wretched condition. He is nauseated, his tongue is coated, he is suffering from headache and from a multitude of other symptoms according to his individual condition. In fact, many of the old aches and pains which he thought already cured come up again with renewed force.

Healing crises, representing radical changes in the system, are always accompanied by physical and mental weakness, because every bit of vitality is drawn upon in these reconstructive processes. The entire organism is shaken up to its very foundation; deep-seated, chronic disease taints are being stirred up throughout the system.

The eliminative processes of the healing crises are often accompanied by great mental depression and a feeling of strong revulsion to the natural regimen and everything connected with it.

The patient thinks that, after all, Nature Cure is not for him, that he is growing worse instead of better. In proportion to the severity of the changes going on within him, he becomes disheartened and despondent. Often he exhibits all the mental and emotional symptoms of homesickness. In these critical days it requires all our powers of persuasion to keep the depressed and discouraged patient from giving up the fight and from taking something to relieve his distress. He insists that "something must be done for him," and cannot understand how he will ever get out of his "awful condition" without some good strong medicine.

If our patients were not continually and thoroughly instructed regarding the Laws of Crises and of Periodicity and if we did not strongly advise and encourage them to persevere with the treatment, few of them would hold out during these critical periods.

This explains why so many people fail to be cured and it also explains why natural living and self-treatment often do not meet with the desired results if carried on without the instruction and guidance of a competent, experienced Nature Cure physician.

So long as the improvement continues, everything is lovely and hope soars high. But when the inevitable crises arrive, the sufferer believes that, after all, he made a mistake in taking up the natural regimen, especially so when friends and relatives do their best to destroy his confidence in the natural methods of cure by ridicule and dire prophesies of failure.

Frightened and discouraged, the patient returns to the "flesh-pots of Egypt" and to the good old pills and potions and ever afterwards he tells his friends that "he tried Nature Cure and the vegetarian diet, but it was no good."

Mother Nature remains a "book sealed with seven seals" to those who mistrust, despise and counteract her, who rely on man-made wisdom and the ever-changing theories and dogmas of the schools.

But on the other hand, every crisis conducted to a successful termination in accordance with Nature's laws becomes an inspiration to him who follows her guidance and assists her with intelligent effort and loving care.

Chapter XXII

What About The "Chronic"?

It Takes So Long

"Yes, Nature Cure is all right, but it takes so long." Now and then we hear this or a similar remark. Our answer is: "No, it does not take long. It is the swiftest cure in existence."

The trouble is that, as a rule, **we have to deal with none but the most advanced cases** of so-called incurable diseases. People go to the Nature Cure physician only after all other methods of treatment have been tried and found of no avail.

As long as there remains a particle of faith in the medicine bottle, the knife or the metaphysical formula of the mind healer, people prefer these easy methods, which require no effort on their part, to the Nature Cure treatment, which necessitates personal exertion, self-control, the changing or giving up of cherished habits. This, however, is what most of us evade as long as we can. "Exercise, the cold blitzguss, no red meat, no coffee?—I'd rather die!"

Afraid of Cold Water

The most-dreaded terror on the threshold seems to be cold water. Undoubtedly, it has kept away thousands from Nature Cure and thereby from the only possible cure for their chronic ailments. If we could achieve equally good results without our heroic methods of treatment, the sidewalks leading to our institution would be crowded with people clamoring for admission.

After all, this foolish fear is entirely groundless. Cold water is no more to be dreaded than the bogey man. It is one of our fundamental principles of treatment never to do anything that is painful to the patient. We always "temper the wind to the shorn lamb," the coldness of the water and the force of the manipulations to the sensitiveness and endurance of the subject. Beginning with mild, alternately warm and cool sprays, which are pleasant and agreeable to everyone, we gradually increase the force and lower the temperature until the patient is so inured to cold water that the blitzguss becomes a delightful and pleasurable sensation, a positive luxury.

It is amusing to watch the gradual change in the attitude of our patients toward the cold-water treatment. In some instances we have had to spend hours in earnest persuasion before we could induce a particularly sensitive person to try the first mild spray. A few weeks later if, perchance, something interfered with the cold water applications, the patient would indignantly refuse to take the other treatment if there was to be no cold water.

There is certainly no finer tonic than cold water, no more exhilarating sensation than that produced by the artistic application of alternating douches and the blitz.

The real cause of this cold-water scare, we believe, is to be found in the boasting of the veterans. When, with protruding chest and chin in air, they brag to the newcomers or to their friends about their heroism and the coolness with which they allow the cold-water hose to be turned on them, the listener shudders and exclaims: "This cold water may be all right for you, but it would never do for me."

No doubt, it is this bravado of the initiated that keeps many a novice from the first plunge into the mysteries of Nature Cure. If these timid ones only knew what they miss!

Business Versus Cure

From a business point of view it would, perhaps, be better to omit the cold water altogether. It would certainly be much less trouble; but then, the rugged honesty of Father Kneipp, the champion of the cold-water treatment branch of German Nature Cure, has descended upon his followers and compels them to tell the whole truth and nothing but the truth, **to make use of everything that is likely to be of benefit to the patient and to effect a real and lasting cure.**

Our friends, the osteopaths, have only a pitying smile for our arduous labors. They ask: "Why fool with cold water and drive patients away, when pleasant manipulations bring the business?" If we query in return: "Do your pleasant manipulations cure obstinate chronic ailments?" They answer: "We do not expect to cure them. The effort involves too much labor and spoils the reputation of our work. Not one in a hundred chronics has the patience and perseverance to be cured. Besides, if a patient comes too long to the office for treatment he drives others away."

Some of the most successful osteopaths in this city make it a rule not to treat a patient longer than six weeks or two months.

In a number of cases this may be sufficient to produce marked primary improvement, but it is not enough to launch the patient into a healing crisis and, therefore, does not produce a **real** cure because it does not remove the underlying causes of the disease. If, after a while, the latent chronic condition again manifests in external symptoms, the patient returns for another course of treatment; he was "cured" so quickly before and thinks he will be helped again.

In justice to the osteopaths it must be said that we are not referring to those chronic diseases which are directly caused by lesions of the spine or other bony structures. If such dislocations or subluxations be the sole cause of the trouble, their correction by manipulative treatment may produce a cure within a few weeks.

But notwithstanding the teachings of orthodox osteopathy, the majority of chronic ailments have their origin in other causes. In most cases, the existing spinal lesions are themselves the result of other primary disease conditions which must be removed before the bony lesions will **remain corrected.**

The mode of treatment depends upon the object that is to be accomplished. If it is to make the patient feel better with the least possible expenditure of time, money, personal effort and self-control on his part, and the least amount of exertion on the part of the physician or healer, then osteopathic manipulations or metaphysical formulas may be in order. But if the object is to cure actually and permanently a deep-seated chronic disease, all the methods of the natural treatment, intelligently combined and adapted to the individual case, will be required in order to accomplish results.

Pull the Roots

Cutting off their heads does not kill the weeds. The first sign of improvement in the treatment of a chronic disease does not mean a cure.

Diagnosis from the Eye, borne out by everyday practical experience, reveals the fact that symptomatic manifestations of disease are due to underlying constitutional causes; that the chronic symptoms are Nature's feeble and ineffectual efforts to eliminate from the system scrofulous, psoric or syphilitic taints and the disease products resulting from food and drug poisoning, or to overcome the destructive effects of surgical mutilations.

An abatement of symptoms is, therefore, not always the sign of a real and permanent cure. The latter depends entirely on the elimination of the hereditary and acquired constitutional taints and poisons.

When, under the influence of natural living and methods of treatment, the body of the chronic becomes sufficiently purified and strengthened, a period of marked improvement may set in. All disease symptoms gradually abate, the patient gains in strength, both physically and mentally, and he feels as though there was nothing the matter with him any more.

But the eyes tell a different story. They show that the underlying constitutional taints have not been fully eliminated—the weeds have not been pulled up by the roots.

This can be accomplished only by healing crises, by Nature's cleansing and healing activities in the form of inflammatory and feverish processes; **anything short of this is merely preliminary improvement,** "training for the fight," **but not the cure.**

When you order a suit of clothes from your tailor, you do not take it away from him half-finished; if you do, you will have an unsatisfactory garment.

No more should you interfere with your cure after the first signs of improvement. Continue until you have thoroughly eliminated from your system the hidden constitutional taints and the drug poisons which have been the cause of your troubles. After that you can paddle your own canoe; right living and right thinking will then be sufficient to maintain perfect health and strength, physically, mentally and morally.

Is the Chronic Patient to Be Left to His Fate Because Allopathy Says He Is Incurable?

Frequently we have been severely criticised by our friends, our co-workers or our patients for accepting certain seemingly hopeless chronic cases. They exclaim:

"You know this man has locomotor ataxy and that woman is an epileptic: you certainly do not expect to cure them," or, "Doctor, don't you think it injures the institution to have that dreadful-looking person around? He is nothing but skin and bones and surely cannot live much longer."

Sometimes open criticism and covert insinuation intimate that our reasons for taking in incurables are mercenary.

If we should dismiss today those of our patients who, from the orthodox and popular point of view, are considered incurable, there would not remain ten out of a hundred; and yet our total failures are few and far between. Many such seemingly hopeless cases have come for treatment month after month, in several instances for a year or more, apparently without any marked advance; yet today they are in the best of health.

Yes, it is hard work and frequently thankless work to deal with these patients. It would be much easier, much more remunerative and would bring more glory to confine ourselves to the treatment of acute diseases, for it is there that Nature Cure works its most impressive miracles. On the other hand, to achieve the seemingly impossible, to prove what Nature Cure can accomplish in the most stubborn chronic cases, sustains our courage and is its own compensation.

The word chronic in the vocabulary of the "Old School" of medicine is synonymous with "incurable." This is not strange; since the medical and surgical symptomatic treatment of acute diseases creates the chronic conditions, it certainly cannot be expected to cure them. If, by continued suppression, Nature's cleansing and healing efforts have been perverted into chronic disease conditions, the following directions are given in the regular works on medical practice:

"When this disease reaches the chronic stage, you can no longer cure it. You may advise the patient to change climate or occupation. As for medication, treat the symptoms as they arise."

We know that the symptoms are Nature's healing efforts; when these are promptly treated, that is, suppressed, it is not surprising that the chronic does not recover. In fact, **it is the treatment which makes him and keeps him a chronic.**

Why Nature Cure Achieves Results

Nature Cure achieves results in the treatment of chronic diseases because its theories and practices are entirely opposite to those just described. However, when the Nature Cure physician claims that he can cure cancer, tuberculosis, epilepsy, paralysis, Bright's disease, diabetes or certain mental derangements, the regular physician shows only derision and contempt. He will not even condescend to examine any evidence in support of our claims.

Since, then, Nature Cure offers to the so-called incurable the only hope and the only possible means of regaining health, why not give him a chance? Many times apparently hopeless cases have responded most readily to our treatment, while more promising ones offered the most stubborn resistance. Even with the best possible methods of diagnosis, it is hard to determine just how far the destruction of vital organs has progressed, or how deeply they have been impregnated with drug poisons.

Therefore, it is often an impossibility to predict with certainty just what the outcome will be. This can be determined only by a fair trial. In the past we have treated many a case that, according to the rules and precedents of orthodox science, should be dead and buried long ago; yet these individuals are today alive and in the best of health.

Every now and then incidents like the following renew our enthusiasm and our faith in Nature Cure: Recently, we had three new cases, sent by three former patients who had been under treatment several years ago. These three had been among the worst cases ever treated in our institution. When they came to us, one was supposed to be dying with cancer, the second was in the advanced stages of tertiary syphilis and the third, a lady, had survived several operations for the removal of the appendix and the ovaries. At the time she took up our treatment she had been advised to undergo another operation for the removal of the uterus.

These incurables had been exceedingly trying. More than once one or another had quit, discouraged and disgusted, only to return, knowing that, after all, Nature Cure was their only hope. After they left us, we lost track of them and often wondered how they were getting on. Imagine our pleasant surprise when all three were reported by the newcomers as being in good health. What if it did take months or even years to produce the desired results? What would have been the fate of these three patients if it had not been for slow Nature Cure?

Discouraged patients frequently ask: "Why do others recover so quickly when I show so little improvement? This cure seems to be all right for some diseases, but evidently it does not fit my case."

This is defective reasoning. True Nature Cure fits every case because it includes everything good in natural healing methods. **In stubborn cases Nature Cure is not to blame for the slow and unsatisfactory results: the difficulty lies in the character and advanced stage of the disease.**

Chapter XXIII

The Treatment of Chronic Diseases

Let us now consider the best methods for producing the healing crises referred to in the preceding chapters, that is, the best methods for treating the chronic forms of disease.

We found that **acute** diseases represent Nature's efforts to purify and regenerate the human organism by means of inflammatory feverish processes, while in the chronic condition the system is not capable of arousing itself to such acute reactions. The treatment must differ accordingly.

The Nature Cure treatment of acute diseases tends to relieve inner congestion, to facilitate the radiation of heat and the elimination of morbid matter and systemic poisons from the body. In this way it eases and palliates the feverish processes and keeps them below the danger point without in any way checking or suppressing them.

While our methods of treating acute diseases have a **sedative** effect, our treatment of chronic diseases is calculated to stimulate, that is, to arouse the sluggish organism to greater activity in order to produce the acute inflammatory reactions or healing crises.

If the unity of diseases as demonstrated in a previous chapter is a fact in Nature, **it must be possible to treat all chronic as well as all acute diseases by uniform methods,** and the natural remedies must correspond to the primary causes of disease.

The Natural Methods of Treatment

Natural methods of treatment may be divided into two groups:

1. Those which the patient can apply himself, provided he has been properly instructed in their correct selection, combination and application.

2. Those which must be applied by a competent Nature Cure physician.

To the first group belong **diet** (fasting), **bathing** and other water applications, **correct breathing,** general **physical exercise, corrective gymnastics, air and sun baths, mental therapeutics.**

To the second group belong special applications of the methods mentioned under group 1, and in addition to these **hydropathy, massage, manipulation, medical treatment** in the form of homeopathic medicines, nonpoisonous herb extracts and the vitochemical remedies, and most important of all, **the right management of healing crises** which develop under the natural treatment of chronic diseases.

Diagnosis

Correct diagnosis is the first essential to rational treatment. Every honest physician admits that the "Old School" methods of diagnosis are, to say the least, unsatisfactory and uncertain, especially in ascertaining the **underlying causes of disease.**

Therefore we should welcome any and all methods of diagnosis which throw more light on the causes and the nature of disease conditions in the human organism.

Two valuable additions to diagnostic science are now offered to us in **osteopathy** and in the **Diagnosis from the Eye.**

Osteopathy furnishes valuable information concerning the connection between disease conditions and misplacements of vertebrae and other bony structures, contractions or abnormal relaxation of muscles and ligaments, and inflammation of nerves and nerve centers.

The Diagnosis from the Eye is as yet a new science, and much remains to be discovered and to be better explained. We do not claim that Nature's records in the eye disclose all the details of pathological tendencies and changes, but they do reveal many disease conditions, hereditary and acquired, that cannot be ascertained by any other methods of diagnosis.

Omitting consideration of everything that is at present speculative and uncertain, we are justified in making the following statements:

1. The eye is not only, as the ancients said, "the mirror of the soul," but it also reveals abnormal conditions and changes in every part and organ of the body.

2. Every organ and part of the body is represented in the iris of the eye in a well-defined area.

3. The iris of the eye contains an immense number of minute nerve filaments, which through the optic nerves, the optic brain centers and the spinal cord are connected with and receive impressions from every nerve in the body.

4. The nerve filaments, muscle fibers and minute blood vessels in the different areas of the iris reproduce the changing conditions in the corresponding parts or organs.

5. By means of various marks, signs, abnormal colors and discolorations in the iris, Nature reveals transmitted disease taints and hereditary lesions.

6. Nature also makes known, by signs, marks and discolorations, acute and chronic inflammatory or catarrhal conditions, local lesions, destruction of tissues, various drug poisons and changes in structures and tissues caused by accidental injury or by surgical mutilations.

7. The Diagnosis from the Eye positively confirms Hahnemann's theory that all acute diseases have a constitutional background of hereditary or acquired disease taints.

8. (This science enables the diagnostician to ascertain, from the appearance of the iris alone, the patient's inherited or acquired tendencies toward health and toward disease, his condition in general and the state of every organin particular. Reading Nature's records in the eye, he can predict the different healing crises through which the patient will have to pass on the road to health.

9. The eye reveals dangerous changes in vital parts and organs from their inception, thus enabling the patient to avert any threatening disease by natural living and natural methods of treatment.

10. By changes in the iris, the gradual purification of the system, the elimination of morbid matter and poisons, and the readjustment of the organism to normal conditions under the regenerating influences of natural living and treatment are faithfully recorded.

This interesting subject will be treated more fully in a separate volume (*Iridiagnosis,* published in 1919 by Dr. Lindlahr). In this connection I shall confine myself to relating briefly the story of the discovery of this valuable science.

The Story of a Great Discovery

Dr. Von Peckzely, of Budapest, Hungary, discovered Nature's records in the eye, quite by accident, when a boy ten years of age.

Playing one day in the garden at his home, he caught an owl. While struggling with the bird, he broke one of its limbs. Gazing straight into the owl's large, bright eyes, **he noticed, at the moment when the bone snapped, the appearance of a black spot in the lower central region of the iris,** which area he later found to correspond to the location of the broken leg.

The boy put a splint on the broken limb and kept the owl as a pet. As the fracture healed, he noticed that the black spot in the iris became overdrawn with a white film and surrounded by a white border (denoting the formation of scar tissues in the broken bone).

This incident made a lasting impression on the mind of the future doctor. It often recurred to him in later years. From further observations he gained the conviction that abnormal physical conditions are portrayed in the eyes.

As a student, Von Peckzely became involved in the revolutionary movement of 1848 and was put in prison as an agitator and ringleader. During his confinement, he had plenty of time and leisure to pursue his favorite theory and he became more and more convinced of the importance of his discovery. After his release, he entered upon the study of medicine, in order to develop his important discoveries and to confirm them more fully in the operating and dissecting rooms. He had himself enrolled as an interne in the surgical wards of the college hospital. Here he had ample opportunity to observe the eyes of patients before and after accidents and operations, and in that manner he was enabled to elaborate the first accurate Chart of the Eye.

Since Von Peckzely gave his discoveries to the world, many well-known scientists and conscientious observers in Austria, Germany and Sweden have devoted their lives to the perfection of this wonderful science. The regular schools of medicine, as a body, have ignored and will ignore it, because it discloses the fallacy of their favorite theories and practices, and because it reveals unmistakably the direful results of chronic drug poisoning and ill-advised operations.

In our work **we do not confine ourselves to the Diagnosis from the Eye,** but combine with it the diagnostic methods (physical diagnosis) of the regular school of medicine and the osteopathic diagnosis of bony lesions, as well as microscopic examinations and chemical analyses.

Thus any one of these methods supplements and verifies all the others. In this way only is it possible to arrive at a thorough and definite understanding of the patient's condition.

Chapter XXIV

Vitality

In Chapter Four, we named, as the first of the primary causes of disease, **lowered vitality.**

What can we do to increase vitality? "Old School" physicians and people in general seem to think that this can be done by consuming large quantities of nourishing food and drink and by the use of stimulants and tonics.

The constant cry of patients is: "Doctor, if you could only prescribe some good tonic or some food that will give me strength, then I should be all right! I am sure that is all I need to be cured."

We fully agree with the patient that he needs more vitality to overcome disease, but unfortunately this cannot be obtained from food and drink, from stimulants and tonics.

Vitality, life, life force, whatever we may call it or whatever its aspect, is not something we can eat and drink. It is independent of the physical body and of material food. If the body should "fall dead," as we call it, the life force would continue to act just as vigorously in the spiritual body, which is the exact counterpart of the physical organism.

The physical-material body as well as the spiritual-material body are only the instruments for the manifestation of the life force. They are no more life itself than the violin is the artist.

But just as the violin must be kept in good condition in order to enable the artist to draw from it the harmonies of sound, so food and drink are necessary to keep the physical body in the best possible condition for the manifestation of vital force. The more normal our physical and spiritual bodies are in structure and function, the more harmonious our thought life and emotional life, the more abundant will be the influx of vital force into the twofold organism.

This important subject has been treated more fully in Chapter IV.

Ignorance of these simple truths leads to the most serious mistakes. Physicians and people in general do not stop to think that excessive eating and drinking tend to **rob** the body of vitality **instead of supplying it.**

The processes of digestion, assimilation and elimination of food and drink in themselves require a considerable expenditure of vital force. Therefore all food taken in excess of the actual needs of the body consumes life force that should be available for other purposes, for the execution of physical and mental work.

The Romans had a proverb: *"Plenus venter non studet libenter"*— "A full stomach does not like to study." The most wholesome food, if taken in excess, will clog the system with waste matter just as too much coal will dampen and extinguish the fire in the furnace.

Furthermore, the morbid materials and systemic poisons produced by impure, unsuitable or wrongly combined foods will clog the cells and tissues of the body, cause unnecessary friction and obstruct the inflow and the operations of the vital energies, just as dust in a watch will clog and impede the movements of its mechanism.

The greatest artist living cannot draw harmonious sounds from the strings of the finest Stradivarius if the body of the violin is filled with dust and rubbish. Likewise, the life force cannot act perfectly in a body filled with morbid encumbrances.

The human organism is capable of liberating and manifesting daily a limited quantity of vital force, just as a certain amount of capital in the bank will yield a specified sum of interest in a given time. If more than the available interest be withdrawn, the capital in the bank will be decreased and gradually exhausted.

Similarly, if we spend more than our daily allowance of vital force, "nervous bankruptcy," that is, nervous prostration or neurasthenia will be the result.

It is the duty of the physician to regulate the expenditure of vital force according to the income. He must stop all leaks and guard against wastefulness.

Stimulation by Paralysis

This heading may seem paradoxical, but it is borne out by fact. Stimulants are poison to the system. Few people realize that their exhilarating and apparently tonic effects are produced by the paralysis of an important part of the nervous system.

If, as we have learned, **wholesome food and drink** in themselves do not contain and therefore **cannot convey life force to the human body, much less can this be accomplished by stimulants.**

The human body has many correspondences with a watch. Both have a motor or driving mechanism and an inhibitory or restraining apparatus.

If it were not for the inhibiting balances, the wound watchspring would run off and spend its force in a few moments. The expenditure of the latent force in the wound spring must be regulated by the inhibitory and balancing mechanism of the timepiece.

Similarly, the nervous system in the animal and human organism consists of two main divisions: the motor or driving and the inhibitory or restraining mechanisms.

The driving power is furnished by the sympathetic nerves and the motor nerves. They convey the vital energies and nerve impulses to the cells and organs of the body, thus initiating and regulating their activities.

We found that the human body is capable of liberating in a given time, say, in twenty-four hours, only a certain limited amount of vital energy, just as the wound spring of the watch is capable of liberating in a given time only a certain amount of kinetic energy.

As in the watch the force of the spring is controlled by the regulating balances (the anchor), so **in the body the expenditure of vital energy must be regulated** in such a manner that it is evenly distributed over the entire running time. **This is accomplished by the inhibitory nervous system** [the parasympathetics].

Every motor nerve must be balanced by an inhibitory nerve. The one furnishes the driving force, the other applies the brake. For instance, the heart muscle is supplied with motor force through the spinal nerves from the upper dorsal region, while the pneumogastric [vagus] nerve retards the action of the heart and in that way acts as a brake.

Another brake is supplied by the waste products of metabolism in the system, the uric acid, carbonic acid, oxalic acid, etc., and the many forms of xanthines, alkaloids, and ptomaines. As these accumulate in the organism during the hours of wakeful activity, they gradually clog the capillary circulation, benumb brain and nerves, and thus produce a feeling of exhaustion and tiredness and a craving for rest and sleep.

In this way, by means of the inhibitory nervous system and of the accumulating fatigue products in the body, Nature forces the organism to rest and recuperate when the available supply of vital force runs low. The lower the level of vital force, the more powerful will become the inhibitory influences.

Now we can understand why stimulation is produced by paralysis. **Stimulants precipitate the fatigue products from the circulation into the tissues of the body.** They do this by overcoming and paralyzing the power of the blood to dissolve and carry in solution uric acid and other acids and alkaloids that should be eliminated from the organism.Thus will be explained more fully in the volume on "Natural Dietetics."

Furthermore, **stimulants temporarily benumb and paralyze the inhibitory nervous system.** In other words, they lift the brakes from the motor nervous system, and allow the driving powers to run wild when Nature wanted them to slow up or stop.

To illustrate: A man has been working hard all day. Toward night his available supply of vitality has run low, his system is filled with uric acid, carbonic acid and other benumbing fatigue products, and he feels tired and sleepy, At this juncture he receives word that he must sit up all night with a sick relative. In order to brace himself for the extraordinary demand upon his vitality, our friend takes a cup of strong coffee, or a drink of whisky, or whatever his favorite stimulant may be.

The effect is marvelous. The tired feeling disappears, and he feels as though he could remain awake all night without effort.

What has produced this apparent renewal and increase of vital energy? Has the stimulant added to his system one iota of vitality? This cannot be, because stimulants do not contain anything that could impart vital force to the organism. What, then, has produced the seemingly strengthening effect?

The caffeine, alcohol or whatever the stimulating poison may have been has precipitated the fatigue products from the blood and deposited them in the tissues and organs of the body. Furthermore, the stimulant has benumbed the inhibitory nerves; in other words, it has lifted the brakes from the driving part of the organism, so that the wheels are running wild.

But this means drawing upon the reserve supplies of nerve fats and of the vital energy stored in them, which Nature wants to save for extraordinary demands upon the system in times of illness or extreme exertion. Therefore this procedure is contrary to Nature's intent. Nature tried to force the tired body to rest and sleep, so that it could store up a new supply of vital force.

Under the paralyzing influence of the stimulant upon the inhibitory nerves, the organism now draws upon the reserve stores of nerve fats and vital energies for the necessary strength to accomplish the extra nightwork.

At the same time, the organism remains awake and active during the time it should be replenishing energy **for the next day's work,** which means that the latter also has to be done at the expense of the reserve supply of life force.

During sleep only do we replenish our reserve stores of vi-

tality. The expenditure of vital energies ceases, but their liberation in the system continues.

Therefore sleep is the "sweet restorer." Nothing can take its place. No amount of food and drink, no tonics or stimulants can make up for the loss of sleep. Continued complete deprivation of sleep is bound to end in a short time in physical and mental exhaustion, in insanity and death.

That the body, during sleep, acts as a storage battery for vital energy is proved by the fact that **in deep, sound sleep the aura disappears entirely from around the body.**

The aura is to the organism what the exhaust steam is to the engine. It is formed by the electromagnetic fluids which have performed their work in the body and then escape from it, giving the appearance of a many-colored halo.

With the first awakening of conscious mental activity after sleep, the aura appears, indicating that the expenditure of vital force has recommenced.

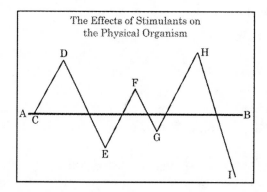

In the above diagram we have an illustration of the true effect of stimulants upon the system. The heavy line A-B represents the normal level of available vital energy in a certain body for a given time, say, for twenty-four hours. At point C a stimulant is taken. This paralyzes the inhibitory nerves and temporarily precipitates the fatigue products from the blood.

As we have seen, this allows an increased, unnatural expenditure of vital energy, which raises the latter to point D. But when the effect of the stimulant has been spent, the vital energy drops from the artificially attained high point not only back to the normal level, but below it to point E.

The increased expenditure of vital energy was made possible at the expense of the reserve supply of vitality; therefore the depression following it is in proportion to the preceding stimulation. This is in accordance with the law: "Action and reaction are equal, but opposite."

The falling of the vital energy **below the normal** to point E is accompanied by a feeling of exhaustion and depression which creates a desire to repeat the pleasurable experience of an abundant supply of vitality, and thus leads to a repetition of the artificial stimulation. As a result of this, the expenditure of vitality is again raised above the normal to point F, only to fall again below the normal, to G, etc.

In this way the person who resorts to stimulants to keep up his strength or to increase it, is never normal, never on the level, never at his best. He is either overstimulated or abnormally depressed. His efforts are bound to be fitful and his work uneven in quality. Furthermore, it will be only a matter of time until he exhausts his reserve supply of nerve fats and vital energy and then suffers nervous bankruptcy in the forms of nervous prostration, neurasthenia or insanity.

Such a person is acting like the spendthrift whose capital in the bank allows him to expend ten dollars a day, but who, instead, draws several times the amount of his legitimate daily interest. There can be but one outcome to this: in due time the cashier will inform him that his account is overdrawn.

The same principles hold true with regard to stimulants given at the sickbed.

One of the arguments I constantly hear from students and physicians of the "Old School" of medicine is: "Some of your methods may be all right, but what would you do at the sickbed of a patient who is so weak and low that he may die at any moment? Would you just let him die? Would you not give him something to keep him alive?"

I certainly would, if I could. But I do not believe that poisons can give life. If there is enough vitality in that dying body to react to the poisonous stimulant by a temporary increase of vital activity, then that same amount of vitality will keep the heart beating and the respiration going a little longer at the slower pace. Nature regulates the heartbeat and the other functions according to the amount and availability of vital force. If the heart beats slow, it is because Nature is trying to economize vitality.

In the inevitable depression following the artificial whipping up of the vital energies, many times the flame is snuffed out entirely when otherwise it might have continued to burn at the slower rate for some time longer.

However, I do not deny the advisability of administering stimulants in cases of shock. When a shock has caused the stopping of the wheels of life, another shock by a stimulant may set them in motion again.

The Effects of Stimulants upon the Mind

The mental and emotional exhilaration accompanying the indulgence in alcohol or other poisonous stimulants is produced in a similar manner as the apparent increase of physical strength under the influence of these agents. **Here, also, the temporary stimulation and seeming increase of power are effected by paralysis of the governing and restraining faculties of mind and soul:** of reason, modesty, reserve, caution, reverence, etc.

The moral, mental and emotional capacities and powers of the human entity are governed by the same principle of dual action that controls physical activity. We have on the one hand the motor or driving impulses, and on the other hand the restraining and inhibiting influences.

In these higher realms appetite, passion, imagination and desire correspond to the motor nervous system in the physical organism, and the power of the will and the reasoning faculties represent the inhibitory nervous system.

The exhilarating and stimulating influence of alcohol and narcotics such as opiates or hashish upon the animal spirits and the emotional and imaginative faculties is caused by the benumbing and paralyzing effect of these stimulants upon the powers of will, reason and self-control, the brakes on the lower appetites, passions and desires which fire the emotional nature and the imagination. However, what is gained in feeling and imagination, is lost in judgment and logic.

Alcohol, nicotine, caffein, theobromine, lupulin (the bitter principle of hops), opium, cocaine, morphine, etc., when given in certain doses, all affect the human organism in a similar manner.

In small quantities they seemingly stimulate and animate; in larger amounts they depress and stupefy. **In reality, they are paralyzers from the beginning in every instance,** and their apparent, temporary tonic effect is deceptive. They benumb and paralyze not only the physical organism, but also the higher and highest mental and moral qualities, capacities and powers.

These higher and finer qualities are located in the front part of the brain. In the evolution of the species from lower to higher, the brain gradually developed and enlarged in a forward direction. Thus we find in the lowest order of fishes that all they possess of brain matter is a small protuberance at the end of the spinal cord. As the species and families rose in the scale of evolution, the brain developed proportionately from behind forward and became differentiated into three distinct divisions: **the medulla oblongata, the cerebellum, and the cerebrum.**

The medulla oblongata, situated at the base of the brain where it joins the spinal cord, contains those brain centers that control the purely vegetative, vital functions: the circulation of the blood, the respiration, regulation of animal heat, etc.

The cerebellum, in front of and above the medulla, is the seat of the centers for the coordination of muscular activities and for maintaining the equilibrium of the body.

The frontal brain or cerebrum contains the centers for the sensory organs, also the motor centers which supply the driving impulses for the muscular activities of the body, and in the occipital and frontal lobes, the centers for the higher and highest qualities of mind and soul, which constitute the governing and restraining faculties on which depend the powers of self-control.

Thus we see that the development of the brain has been in a forward direction, from the upper extremity of the spinal cord to the frontal lobes of the cerebrum, from the low, vegetative qualities of the animal and the savage to the complex and refined activities of the highly civilized and trained mind.

It is an interesting and most significant fact that **paralysis of brain centers caused by alcohol and other stimulants, or by hypnotics and narcotics, proceeds reversely to the order of their development during the processes of evolution.**

The first to succumb are the brain centers in the frontal lobes of the cerebrum, which control the latest-developed and most-refined human attributes. These are: **modesty, caution, reserve, reverence, altruism.** Then follow in the order given: **memory, reason, logic, intelligence, will power, self-control,** the **control of muscular coordination** and **equilibrium** and finally **consciousness** and the vital activities of **heart action** and **respiration.**

When the conscious activities of the soul have been put to sleep, the paralysis extends to the subconscious activities of life or vital force. Respiration and heart action become weak and labored, and may finally cease entirely.

In order to verify this, let us study the effects of **alcohol,** the best-known and most-used of stimulants. Many people believe that alcohol increases not only physical strength, but mental energy also. Regular medical science considers it a valuable tonic in all cases of physical and mental depression. It is often administered in surgical operations and in accidents with the idea of prolonging life. I have frequently found the whisky or brandy bottle at the bedside of infants and on it the directions of the attending physician.

Watch the effect of this tonic on a group of convivial spirits at a banquet. Full honor is done to the art of the chef, and the wine flows freely. The flow of animal spirits increases proportionately; conviviality, wit and humor rise by leaps and bounds. But the apparent joy and happiness are in reality nothing but the play of the lower animal impulses, unrestrained by the higher powers of mind and soul.

The words of the afterdinner speaker who, when sober, is a sedate and earnest gentleman, flow with unusual ease. The close and unprejudiced observer notices, however, that what the speaker has gained in eloquence, loquacity and exuberance of style and expression, he has lost in logic, clearness and good sense.

As King Alcohol tightens his grasp on the merry company, the toasters and speakers lose more and more their control over speech and actions. What was at first mischievous abandon and merry jest, gradually degenerates into loquaciousness, coarseness and querulous brawls. Here and there one of the maudlin crowd drops off in the stupor of drunkenness.

If the liquor is strong enough and if the debauch is continued long enough, it may end in complete paralysis of the vital functions or in death.

Hypnotism and Obsession

Again, we find the seeming paradox of stimulation by paralysis exemplified in the phenomena of hypnotism and obsession. **The abnormally exaggerated sensation, feeling and imagination of the subject under hypnotic control are made possible because the higher, critical and restraining faculties and powers of will, reason and self-control are temporarily or permanently benumbed and paralyzed** by the stronger will of the hypnotist or of the obsessing intelligence.

There is a most interesting resemblance between the effects of stimulants, narcotics or hypnotic control and blind, unreasoning faith. The latter also benumbs and paralyzes judgment and reason. It gives full sway to the powers of imagination and thus may produce seemingly miraculous results.

This explains the modus operandi of faith cures as well as the fitful strength of the intoxicated and the insane, or the beautiful dreams and delusions of grandeur of the drug addict.

The close resemblance and relationship between hypnotic control and faith became vividly apparent to me while witnessing the performance of a professional hypnotist. His subject on the stage was a young woman who, under his control, performed extraordinary feats of strength and resistance. Several strong men could not lift or move her in any way.

What was the reason? In the ordinary, waking condition her judgment and common sense would tell her: "I cannot resist the combined strength of these men. Of course, they can lift me and pull me here and there." As a result of this doubting state of mind, she would not have the strength to resist.

However, the control of the hypnotist had paralyzed her reasoning faculties and therewith her capacity for judging, doubting and not believing. Her subconscious mind accepted without question or the shadow of a doubt the suggestion of the hypnotist that she did possess the strength to resist the combined efforts of the men and as a result she actually manifested the necessary powers of resistance.

It is an established fact that the impressions (records) made upon the subconscious mind under certain conditions as, for instance, under hypnotic influence absolutely control the activities of the physical body.

Does not this throw an interesting light on the power of absolute faith, on the saying: "Everything is possible to him who believeth?" Blind, unreasoning faith benumbs and paralyzes judgment and reason in similar manner as hypnotic control or stimulants and in that way gives free and full sway to the powers of imagination and autosuggestion for good or ill, for white magic or black magic, according to the purpose for which faith is exerted.

It also becomes apparent that such blind, unreasoning faith cannot be constructive in its influence upon the higher mental, moral and spiritual faculties. **These can be developed only by the conscious and voluntary exercise of will, reason and self-control.**

From the foregoing it will have become evident that we cannot increase vital force in the body through any artificial means or methods from without, by food, drink or stimulant. What we can and should do, however, is to put the organism into the best possible condition for the liberation and manifestation of life force or vital energy.

The more normal the chemical composition of the blood, and the more free the tissues are from clogging impurities, poisons and mechanical obstructions, such as lesions of the spinal column, the more abundant will be the liberation and the available supply of vital energy.

Therefore perfect, buoyant health, which ensures the greatest possible efficiency and enjoyment of life, can be attained and maintained only by strict adherence to the natural ways of living and, when necessary, by the natural treatment of diseases.

Chapter XXV

Natural Dietetics

The chemical composition of blood and lymph depends upon the chemical composition of food and drink, and upon the normal or abnormal condition of the digestive organs.

The purer the food and drink, the less it contains of morbid matter and poison-producing materials and the more it contains of the elements necessary for the proper execution of the manifold functions of the organism, for the building and repair of tissues and for the neutralization and elimination of waste and systemic poisons, the more "normal" and the more "natural" will be the diet.

The system of dietetics of the Nature Cure school is based upon the composition of MILK, which is the only perfect natural food combination in existence.

In its composition, milk corresponds very closely to red, arterial blood and contains all the elements which the newborn and growing organism needs in exactly the right proportions, providing, of course, that the human or animal body which produces the milk is in good health and lives on pure and normal foods.

Therefore, if any food combination or diet is to be "normal" or "natural," it must approach in its chemical composition the chemical composition of milk or of red, arterial blood. This furnishes a strictly scientific basis for an exact science of dietetics, and proves true not only in the chemical aspect of the diet problem, but also in every other aspect and in its practical application.

The "regular" school of medicine pays little or no attention to rational food regulation. In fact, it knows nothing about it, because "natural dietetics" are as yet not taught in medical schools. As a result of this condition, the dietary advice given by the majority of Old School practitioners is something as follows: "Eat what agrees with you: plenty of good, nourishing food. There is nothing in dietetic fads. What is one man's meat is another man's poison, etc."

However, if we study dietetics from a strictly scientific point of view, we find that certain foods—among these especially the highly valued flesh foods, eggs, pulses and cereals—create in the system large quantities of morbid, poisonous substances, while on the other hand fruits and vegetables, which are rich in the organic salts, tend to neutralize and to eliminate from the system the waste materials and poisons created in the processes of protein and starch digestion.

The accumulations of waste and systemic poisons are the cause of the majority of diseases arising within the human organism. Therefore it is imperative that the neutralizing and eliminating food elements be provided in sufficient quantities.

On this turns the entire problem of natural dietetics. While the "Old School" of medicine looks upon starches, sugars, fats and proteins as the only elements of nutrition worthy of consideration, **Nature Cure aims to reduce these foods in the natural dietary and to increase the purifying and eliminating fruits and vegetables.**

In this volume we cannot go into the details of the diet question. They will be treated in full in our *Vegetarian Cookbook* and in our volume on *Natural Dietetics*. We shall say here in a general way that **in the treatment of chronic diseases,** with few exceptions, **we favor a strict vegetarian diet** for the reason that most chronic diseases are created, as before stated, by the accumulation of the "feces of the cells" in the system.

Every piece of animal flesh is saturated with these excrements of the cells in the form of uric acid and many other kinds of acids, alkaloids of putrefaction, xanthines, ptomaines, etc. The organism of the meat eater must dispose not only of its own impurities produced in the processes of digestion and of cell metabolism, but also of the morbid substances that are already contained in the animal flesh.

Since the cure of chronic diseases consists largely in purifying the body of morbid materials, it stands to reason that a "chronic" must cease taking these in his daily food and drink. To do otherwise would be like sweeping the dirt out of a house through the front door and carrying it in again through the back door.

Whether one approves of strict vegetarianism as a continuous mode of living or not, it will be admitted that the change from a meat diet to a nonmeat diet must be of great benefit in the treatment of chronic diseases.

The cure of chronic conditions depends upon radical changes in the cells and tissues of the body, as explained in Chapter Twenty. The old, abnormal, faulty diet will continue to build the same abnormal and disease-encumbered tissues. The more thorough and radical the change in diet toward normality and purity, the quicker the cells and tissues of the body will change toward the normal and thus bring about a complete regeneration of the organism.

DIETICS IN A NUTSHELL

	Food Classes	Predominant Chemical Elements	Predominant Chemical Elements	Foods in Which the Elements of the Respective Groups Predominate
GROUP I **Carbohydrates**	Starches and Dextrines	Carbon Oxygen Hydrogen	Producers of Heat and Energy	CEREALS: The inner, white parts of wheat, corn, rye, oats, barley, buckewheat and rice. VEGETABLES: Potatoes, pumpkins, squashes. FRUITS: Bananas. NUTS: Chestnuts
GROUP II **Carbohydrates**	Sugars	Carbon Oxygen Hydrogen	Producers of Heat and Energy	VEGETABLES: Melons, beets, sorghum. FRUITS: Bananas, dates, figs, grapes, raisins. DAIRY PRODUCTS: Milk. NATURAL SUGARS: Honey, maple sugar. COMMERCIAL SUGARS: White sugar, syrup, glucose, candy. NUTS: Cocoanuts.
GROUP III **Hydrocarbons**	Fats and Oils	Carbon Oxygen Hydrogen	Producers of Heat and Energy	FRUITS: Olives. DAIRY PRODUCTS: Cream, butter, cheese. NUTS: Peanuts, almonds, walnuts, cocoanuts, Brazil nuts, pecans, pignolias, etc. COMMERCIAL FATS: Olive oil, peanut oil, peanut butter, vegetable-cooking oils. THE YOKES OF EGGS
GROUP IV **Proteids**	Albumen (white of egg) Gluten (grains) Myosin (lean meat)	Carbon Oxygen Hydrogen Nitrogen Phosphorus Sulphur	Producers of Heat and Energy; Building Materials for Cells and Tissues	CEREALS: The outer, dark parts of wheat, corn, rye, oats, barley, buckwheat, and rice. VEGETABLES: The legumes (peas, beans, lentils), mushrooms. NUTS: Cocoanuts, chestnuts, peanuts, pignolias (pine nuts), hickorynuts, hazelnuts, walnuts, pecans, etc. DAIRY PRODUCTS: Milk, cheese. MEATS: Muscular parts of animals, fish, and fowls.
GROUP V **Organic Minerals**	Organic Mineral Elements	Sodium Na Ferrum (Iron) Fe Calcium (Lime) Ca Potassium K Magnesium Mg Manganese Mn Silicon Si Chlorine Cl Flourine Fl	Eliminators: Bone, Blood, and Nerve Builders; Antiseptics: Blood Purifiers; Laxitives; Cholagogues; Producers of Electromagnetic Energies	THE RED BLOOD OF ANIMALS. CEREALS: The hulls and outer, dark layers of grains and rice. VEGETABLES: Lettuce, spinach, cabbage, green peppers, watercress, celery, onions, asparagus, cauliflower, tomatoes, string-beans, fresh peas, parsley, cucumbers, radishes, savoy, horseradish, dandelion, beets, carrots, turnips, eggplant, kohlrabi, oysterplant, artichokes, leek, rosekale (Brussels sprouts), parsnips, pumpkins, squashes, sorghum. FRUITS: Apples, pears, peaches, oranges, lemons, grapefruit, plums, prunes, apricots, cherries, olives. BERRIES: Strawberries, huckleberries, cranb \erries, blackberries, blueberries, raspberries, gooseberries, currants. DAIRY PRODUCTS: Milk, buttermilk, skimmed milk. NUTS: Cocoanuts.

Anything short of this may be palliative treatment, but is not worthy the name of cure.

Natural Foods

In the following I shall give the outline a natural diet regimen which has been found by experience to meet all requirements of the healthy organism, even when people have to work very hard physically or mentally. In case of disease, certain modifications may have to be made according to individual conditions. Persons in a low, negative state, whether physical, mental or psychical, may temporarily require the addition of flesh foods to their diet.

In the accompanying table entitled "Dietics In A Nutshell" we have divided all food materials into five groups:

GROUP:

1. (Carbohydrates): Starches.
2. (Carbohydrates): Dextrins and sugars.
3. (Hydrocarbons): Fats and oils.
4. (Proteids): white of egg, lean meat, the gluten of grains and pulses, the proteins of nuts and milk.
5. (Organic Minerals): Iron, sodium calcium, potassium, magnesium, silicon. These are contained in largest amounts in the juicy fruits and the leafy, juicy vegetables.

As a general rule, let one-half of your food consist of Group V and the other half of a mixture of the first four groups.

If you wish to follow a pure food diet, exclude meat, fish, fowl, meat soups and sauces and all other foods prepared from the dead animal carcass.

This is brief and comprehensive. When in doubt, consult this rule.

Also do not use coffee, tea, alcoholic beverages, tobacco or stimulants of any kind.

Good foods are:

Dairy Products: milk, buttermilk, skimmed milk, cream, butter, fresh cottage cheese. fermented cheeses, as American, Swiss, Holland and DeBrie, should be used sparingly. The stronger cheeses like Camembert and Roquefort should not be used at all

Eggs: Raw, soft-boiled or poached, not fried or hard-boiled. Eggs should be used sparingly. Two eggs three times a week or on an average one egg a day, is sufficient.

White of egg is much easier to digest than the yolk, therefore the whites only should be used in cases of very weak digestion. Beaten up with orange juice, they are both palatable and wholesome; or they may be beaten very stiff and served cold with a sauce of prune juice or other cooked fruit juices. This makes a delicious and very nutritive dish.

Honey is a very valuable food and a natural laxative. It is not generally known that honey is not a purely vegetable product, but that in passing through the organism of the bee it partakes of its life element (animal magnetism).

Honey is one of the best forms of sugar available. The white sugar is detrimental to health, because it has become inorganic through the refining process. The brown, unrefined granulated sugar or maple sugar should be used instead.

Figs, dates, raisins, bananas and all the other sweet fruits are excellent to satisfy the craving of the organism for sweets.

Cereal Foods: Rice, wheat, oats, barley, are good when properly combined with fruits and vegetables and with dairy products.Use preferably the whole-grain preparations such as shredded wheat or corn flakes. Oatmeal is not easily digestible; it is all right for robust people working in the open air, but not so good for invalids and people of sedentary habits.

Thin mushes are not to be recommended, because they do not require mastication and therefore escape the action of the saliva, which is indispensable to the digestion of starchy foods.

Avoid the use of white bread or any other white-flour products, especially pastry. White flour contains little more than the starchy elements of the grain. Most of the valuable proteins which are equal to meat in food value and the all-important organic salts which lodge in the hulls and the outer layers of the grain have been refined out of it together with the bran. The latter is in itself very valuable as a mechanical stimulant to the peristaltic action of the bowels.

In preference to white bread eat Graham bread or whole rye bread. Our health bread forms the solid foundation of a well-balanced vegetarian diet. It is prepared as follows:

Take one-third each of white flour, Graham flour and rye meal (not the ordinary Bohemian rye flour, but the coarse pumpernickel meal which contains the whole of the rye, including the hull).

Make a sponge of the white flour in the usual manner, either with good yeast or with leavened dough from the last baking, which has been kept cold and sweet. When the sponge has risen sufficiently, work the graham flour and rye meal into it. Thorough kneading is of importance. Let rise slowly a second time, place in pans, and bake slowly until thoroughly done.

By chemical analysis this bread has been found to contain more nourishment than meat. It is very easily digested and assimilated and is a natural laxative. Eaten with sweet butter and in combination with fruits and vegetables, it makes a complete and well balanced meal.

A good substitute for bread is the following excellent whole wheat preparation: Soak clean, soft wheat in cold water for about seven hours and steam in a double boiler for from eight to twelve hours, or cook in a fireless cooker over night. Eat with honey and milk or cream, or with prune juice, fig juice, etc., or add butter and dates or raisins. This dish is more nutritious than meat, and one of the finest laxative foods in existence.

Nuts are exceedingly rich in fats (60 percent) and proteins (15 percent), but rank low in mineral salts. Therefore they should be used sparingly, and always in combination with fruits, berries or vegetables. The coconut differs from the other nuts in that it contains less fats and proteins and more organic salts. The meat of the coconut together with its milk comes nearer to the chemical composition of human milk than any other food in existence.

Vegetables

Leguminous Vegetables, such as peas, beans and lentils in the ripened state are richer in protein than meat (25 percent), and besides they contain a large percentage of starchy food elements (60 percent); therefore they produce in the process of digestion large quantities of poisonous acids, alkaloids of putrefaction and noxious gases.

They should not be taken in large quantities and only in combination cooked or raw vegetables. As a dressing use lemon juice and olive oil.

Peas and beans in the green state differ very much from their chemical composition in the ripened state. As long as these vegetables are green and in the pulp, they contain large quantities of sugars and organic minerals, with but little starch and protein. As the ripening process advances, the percentages of starches and proteins increase, while those of the sugars and of the organic minerals decrease. The latter retire into the leaves and stems (polarization).

In the green, pulpy state these foods may, therefore, be classed with Group II (Sugars) and with Group V (Organic Minerals), while in the ripened state they must be classed with Groups I (Starches) and Groups IV (Proteids).

Dried peas, beans and lentils are more palatable and wholesome when cooked in combination with tomatoes or prunes.

The Leafy and Juicy Vegetables growing in or near the ground are very rich in the **positive** organic salts and therefore of great nutritive and medicinal value. For this reason they are best suited to balance the **negative,** acid-producing starches, sugars, fats and proteins.

Lettuce, spinach, cabbage, watercress, celery, parsley, savoy cabbage, brussels sprouts, Scotch kale, leek and endive rank highest in organic mineral salts. Next to these come tomatoes, cucumbers, green peppers, radishes, onions, asparagus, cauliflower and horseradish.(See also Group V in "Dietetics in a Nutshell.")

Splendid, cooling summer foods, rich in the blood-purifying organic salts, are watermelons, muskmelons. cantaloupes, pumpkins, squashes and other members of the melon family.

The green vegetables are most beneficial when eaten **raw,** with a dressing of lemon juice and olive oil. Avoid the use of vinegar as much as possible. It is a product of fermentation and a powerful preservative which retards digestion as well as fermentation, both processes being very much of the same character.

Use neither pepper nor salt at the table. They may be used sparingly in cooking. Strong spices and condiments are more or less irritating to the mucous linings of the intestinal tract. They paralyze gradually the nerves of taste. At first they stimulate the digestive organs; but, like all other stimulants, in time they produce weakness and atrophy.

Cooking of Vegetables

While most vegetables are not improved by cooking, we do not mean that they should never be cooked. Many diet reformers go to extremes when they claim that all the organic salts in fruits and vegetables are rendered **inorganic** by cooking. This is an exaggeration. Cooking is merely a mechanical process of subdivision, not a chemical process of transformation. Mechanical processes of division do not dissolve or destroy organic molecules to any great extent.

Nevertheless, it remains true that the green leafy vegetables are not improved by cooking. It is different with the starchy tubers and roots like potatoes, turnips, etc., and with other starchy foods such as rice and grains. Here the cooking serves to break up and separate the hard starch granules and to make them more pervious to penetration by the digestive juices.

How to Cook Vegetables

After the vegetables are thoroughly washed and cut into pieces as desired, place them in the cooking vessel, adding only enough water to keep them from burning, cover the vessel closely with a lid and let them steam slowly in their own juices.

The leafy vegetables (cabbage, spinach, kale, etc.), usually contain enough water for their own steaming.

Cook all vegetables only as long as is required to make them soft enough for easy mastication. Do not throw away a drop of the water in which such vegetables as carrots, beets, asparagus, oyster plant, egg plant, etc., have been cooked. Use what is left for the making of soups and sauces.

The organic mineral salts contained in the vegetables readily boil out into the water. If the vegetables, as is the usual custom, are boiled in a large quantity of water, then drained or, what is still worse, pressed out, they have lost their nutritive and medicinal value. The mineral salts have vanished in the sink, the remains are insipid and indigestible and have to be soaked in soup stock and seasoned with strong condiments and spices to make them at all palatable.

Fruits and Berries

Next to the leafy vegetables, fruits and berries are the most valuable foods of the organic minerals group. Lemons, grapefruit, oranges, apples are especially beneficial as blood purifiers. Plums, pears, peaches, apricots, cherries, grapes, etc., contain large amounts of fruit sugars in easily assimilable form and are also very valuable on account of their mineral salts.

The different kinds of berries are even richer in mineral salts than the acid and subacid fruits. In the country homes of Germany they are always at hand either dried or preserved to serve during the winter not only as delicious foods but also as valuable home remedies.

Fruits and berries are best eaten raw, although they may be stewed or baked. Very few people know that rhubarb and cranberries are very palatable when cut up fine and well mixed with honey, being allowed to stand for about an hour before serving. Prepared in this way, they require much less sweetening and therefore do not tax the organism nearly as much as the ordinary rhubarb or cranberry sauce, which usually contains an excessive amount of sugar.

Cooking of Fruits

It is better to cook apples, cranberries, rhubarb, strawberries, and all other acid fruits **without sugar** until soft, and to add the sugar afterward. Much less sugar will be required to sweeten them sufficiently than when the sugar is added before or during the cooking.

Dried fruits rank next to the fresh in value, as the evaporating process only removes a large percentage of water, without changing the chemical composition of the fruit in any way. Prunes, apricots, apples, pears, peaches and berries may be obtained in the dried state all through the year. Dates, figs, raisins and currants also come under this head.

Olives are an excellent food. They are very rich in fats (about 50 percent), and contain also considerable quantities of organic salts. They are therefore a good substitute for animal fat.

Avoid factory-canned fruits. In the first place, they have become deteriorated by the cooking process and secondly, they usually contain poisonous chemical preservatives. Home-preserved fruits and vegetables are all right providing they do not contain too much sugar and no poisonous preservative.

Bananas differ from the juicy fruits in that they consist almost entirely of starches, dextrines and sugars. They belong to the carbohydrate groups and should be used sparingly by people suffering from intestinal indigestion.

However, we do not share the belief entertained by many people that bananas are injurious under all circumstances. We consider them an excellent food, especially for children.

Mixing Fruits and Vegetables

Many people, when they first sit down to our table, are horrified to see how we mix fruits and vegetables in the same meal. They have been taught that it is a cardinal sin against the laws of health to do this. After they overcome their prejudice and partake heartily of the meals as we serve them, they are greatly surprised to find that these combinations of vegetables and juicy fruits are not only harmless, but agreeable and highly beneficial.

We have never been able to find any good reason why these foods should not be mixed and our experience proves that no ill effects can be traced to this practice except in very rare instances. There are a few individuals with whom the mixing of fruits and vegetables does not seem to agree. These, of course, should refrain from it. We must comply with idiosyncrasies until they are overcome by natural living.

Eating fruits only or vegetables only at one and the same meal limits the selection and combination of foods to a very considerable extent and tends to create monotony, which is not only unpleasant but injurious. The flow of saliva and of the digestive juices is greatly increased by the agreeable sight, smell and taste of appetizing food and these depend largely upon its variety.

With very few exceptions, every one of our patients (and we have in our institution as fine a collection of dyspeptics as can be found anywhere) heartily enjoys our mixed dietary and is greatly benefited by it.

Mixing Starches and Acid Fruits

Occasionally we find that one or another of our patients cannot eat starchy foods and acid fruits at the same meal without experiencing digestive disturbances. Whenever this is the case, it is best to take with bread or cereals only sweet, alkaline fruits such as prunes, figs, dates, raisins, or, in their season, watermelons and cantaloupes or the alkaline vegetables such as radishes, lettuce, onions, cabbage slaw, etc. The acid and subacid fruits should then be taken **between** those meals which consist largely of starchy foods.

A Word About the Milk Diet

When we explain that the natural diet is based upon the chemical composition of milk because milk is the only perfect natural food combination in existence, the question comes up: "Why, then, not live on milk entirely?" To this we reply: While milk is the natural food for the newborn and growing infant, it is not natural for the adult. The digestive apparatus of the infant is especially adapted to the digestion of milk, while that of the adult requires more solid and bulky food.

Milk is a very beneficial article of diet in all acid diseases, because it contains comparatively low percentages of carbohydrates and proteins and large amounts of organic salts.

However, not everybody can use milk as a food or medicine. In many instances it causes biliousness, fermentation and constipation.

In cases where it is easily digested, a straight milk diet often proves very beneficial. As a rule, however, it is better to take fruits or vegetable salads with the milk.

Directly with milk may be taken any sweetish, alkaline fruits such as melons, sweet pears, etc., or the dried fruits, such as prunes, dates, figs, and raisins, also vegetable salads. With the latter, if taken together with milk, little or no lemon juice should be used.

All acid and subacid fruits should be taken **between** the milk meals.

A patient on a milk diet may take from one to five quarts of milk daily, according to his capacity to digest it. This quantity may be distributed over the day after the following plan:

Breakfast: One to three pints of milk, sipped slowly with any of the sweetish, alkaline fruits mentioned above, or with vegetable salads composed of lettuce, celery, raw cabbage slaw, watercress, green onions, radishes, carrots, etc

10:00 A.M.: Grapefruit, oranges, peaches, apples, apricots, berries, grapes or other acid and subacid fruits.

Luncheon: The same as breakfast.

3:00 P.M. The same as 10 a.m.

Supper: The same as breakfast. An orange or apple may be taken before retiring.

When it is advisable to take a greater variety of food together with large quantities of milk, good whole grain bread and butter, cream, honey, cooked vegetables, moderate amounts of potatoes and cereals may be added to the dietary.

Buttermilk

Buttermilk is an excellent food for those with whom it agrees. In many instances a straight buttermilk diet for a certain period will prove very beneficial. This is especially true in all forms of uric acid diseases.

Sour milk or clabber also has excellent medicinal qualities and may be taken freely by those with whom it agrees.

Drinks

It has been stated before that coffee, tea and alcoholic beverages should be avoided.

Instead of the customary coffee, tea or cocoa, delicious drinks, which are nutritious and at the same time **nonstimulating**, may be prepared from the different fruit and vegetable juices. They may be served cold in hot weather and warm in winter. Recipes for fruit and vegetable drinks will be included in our new **Vegetarian Cookbook,** now in preparation.

If more substantial drinks are desired, white of egg may be added or the entire egg may be used in combination with prune juice, fig juice or any of the acid fruit juices. Other desirable and unobjectionable additions to beverages are flaked nuts or bananas mashed to a liquid.

The juice of a lemon or an orange, unsweetened, diluted with twice the amount of water, taken upon rising, is one of the best means of purifying the blood and other fluids of the body and, incidentally, clearing the complexion. The water in which prunes or figs have been cooked should be taken freely to remedy constipation.

As a practical illustration, I shall describe briefly the daily dietary regimen as it is followed in our sanitarium work.

Breakfast consists of juicy fruits, raw, baked or stewed, a cereal (whole wheat steamed, cracked wheat, shredded wheat, corn flakes, oat meal, etc.), and our health bread with butter, cottage cheese or honey. Nuts of various kinds, as well as figs, dates, or raisins, are always on the table. To those of our patients who desire a drink, we serve milk, buttermilk or cereal coffee.

Twice a week we serve eggs, preferably raw, soft boiled or poached.

Luncheon is served at noontime and is composed altogether of acid and subacid fruits, vegetable salads or both. We have found by experience that, by having one meal consist entirely of fruits and vegetables, the medicinal properties of these foods have a chance to act on the system without interference by starchy and protein food elements.

Dinner is served to our patients between five and six. The items of the daily menu comprise relishes, such as radishes, celery, olives, young onions, raw carrots, etc., soup, one or two cooked vegetables, potatoes, preferably boiled or baked in their skins, and a dessert consisting of either a fruit combination or a pudding.

We serve soup three times a week only, because we believe that a large amount of fluid of any kind taken into the system at meal time dilutes and thereby weakens the digestive juices. For this reason it is well to masticate with the soup some bread or crackers or some vegetable relish.

As drinks we serve to those who desire it water, milk or buttermilk.

Prunes or figs, stewed or raw, are served at every meal to those who require a specially laxative diet.

Chapter XXVI

Acid Diseases

The origin, progressive development and cure of acid diseases are very much the same whether they manifest as rheumatism, arteriosclerosis, stones (calculi), gravel, diabetes, Bright's disease, affections of the heart or apoplexy.

The human body is made up of acid and alkaline constituents. In order to have normal conditions and functions of tissues and organs, both must be present in the right proportions. If either the acid or the alkaline elements are present in excessive or insufficient quanitities, abnormal conditions and functions, that is, **disease** will be the result.

All acids, with the exception of carbonic acid, **exert a tensing influence** upon the tissues of the body, **while alkalies have a relaxing effect.** The normal functions of the body depend upon the equilibrium between these opposing forces.

Acidity and alkalinity undoubtedly play an important part in the generation of electricity and magnetism in the human organism. Every electric cell and battery contains acid and alkaline elements; and the human body is a dynamo made up of innumerable minute electric cells and batteries in the forms of living, protoplasmic cells and organs.

It has been claimed that what we call vital force is **electricity** and **magnetism,** and that these forces are manufactured in the human body. This, however, is but a partial statement of the truth. It is true that vital force manifests in the body as electricity and magnetism, but life or vital force itself is not generated in the system.

Life is a primary force; it is the source of all activity animating the universe. From this primary force other, secondary forces are derived, such as electricity, magnetism, mind force, nerve and muscle force, etc.

These secondary, derived forces cannot be changed back into vital force in the human organism. Nothing can give life but LIFE itself.

When the physical body is dead, as we call it, the life which left it is active in the spiritual body. It is independent of the physical organism just as electricity is independent of the incandescent bulb in which it manifests as light.

After this digression we shall return to our study of the cause and development of acid diseases. Nearly every disease originating in the human body is due to or accompanied by the excessive formation of different kinds of acids in the system, the most important of which are uric, carbonic, sulphuric, phosphoric and oxalic acids. These, together with xanthines, poisonous alkaloids and ptomaines, are formed during the processes of protein and starch digestion and in the breaking down and decay of cells and tissues.

Of these different waste products, **uric acid** causes probably the most trouble in the organism. The majority of diseases arising within the human body are due to its erratic behavior. Together with oxalic acid, it is responsible for arteriosclerosis, arthritic rheumatism and the formation of calculi.

Dr. Haig of London has done excellent work in the investigation of uric-acid poisoning, but he becomes one-sided when he makes uric acid the scapegoat for all disease conditions originating in the organism. In his philosophy of disease he fails to take into consideration the effects of other acids and systemic poisons. For instance, he does not mention the fact that carbonic acid is produced in the system somewhat similarly to the formation of coal gas in the furnace; and that its accumulation prevents the entrance of oxygen into the cells and tissues, thus causing asphyxiation or oxygen starvation, which manifests in the symptoms of anemia and tuberculosis.

Neither does Dr. Haig explain the effects of other destructive by-products formed during the digestion of starches and proteins. Sulphurous acid and sulphuric acid (vitriol), as well as phosphorus and phosphoric acids **actually burn up the tissues of the body.** They destroy the cellulose membranes which form the protecting skins or envelopes of the cells, dissolve the protoplasm and allow the latter to escape into the circulation. This accounts for the symptoms of Bright's disease, the presence of albumen (cell protoplasm) in blood and urine, the clogging of the circulation, the consequent stagnation and the accumulation of blood serum (dropsy) and the final breaking down of the tissues (necrosis) resulting in open sores and ulcers.

Excess of phosphorus and the acids derived from it overstimulates the brain and the nervous system, causing nervousness, irritability, hysteria and the different forms of mania.

An example of this is the distemper of a horse when given too much oats and not enough grass or hay. The excess of phosphorus and phosphoric acids formed from the protein materials of the grain, if not neutralized by the alkaline minerals contained in grasses, hay or straw, will overstimulate and irritate the nervous system of the animal and cause it to become nervous, irritable and vicious. These symptoms disappear when the rations of oats are decreased and when more fresh grass or hay is fed in place of the grain.

Similar effects to those produced upon the horse by an excess of grains are caused in the human organism, especially in the sensitive nervous system of the child, by a surplus of protein foods, of meat, eggs, grains and pulses.

Still, when patients suffering from overstimulation of the brain and nervous system consult their doctor, his advice in almost every instance is: "Your nerves are weak and overwrought. You need plenty of good, nourishing food (broths, meat and eggs), and 'a good tonic.'"

The remedies prescribed by the doctor are the very things which caused the trouble in the first place.

As stated before, uric acid is undoubtedly one of the most common causes of disease and therefore deserves especial attention. Through the study of its peculiar behavior under different circumstances and influences, the cause, nature and development of all acid diseases will become clearer.

Like urea, uric acid is one of the end products of protein digestion. It is formed in much smaller quantities than urea, in proportion of about one to fifty, but the latter is more easily eliminated from the system through kidneys and skin.

The principal ingredient in the formation of uric acid is **nitrogen,** one of the six elements which enter into all proteid or albuminous food materials, also called nitrogenous foods. Uric acid, as one of the by-products of digestion, is therefore always present in the blood and, in moderate quantities, serves useful purposes in the economy of the human and animal organism like the other waste materials. It becomes a source of irritation and cause of disease only when it is present in the circulation or in the tissues in excessive amounts.

How Uric Acid Is Precipitated

The alkaline blood takes up the uric acid, dissolves it and holds it in solution in the circulation until it is carried to the organs of depuration and eliminated in perspiration and urine. If, however, through the excessive use of nitrogenous foods or defective elimination, **the amount of uric acid in the system is increased beyond a certain limit,** the blood loses its power to dissolve it and it forms a sticky, glue-like, colloid substance, which occludes or blocks up the minute blood vessels (capillaries), so that the blood cannot pass readily from the arterial system into the venous circulation.

This interference with the free passing of the blood is greater in proportion to the distance from the heart, because the farther from the heart, the less the force behind the circulation. Therefore we find that slowing up of the blood currents, whether due to uric acid occlusion or any other cause, is more pronounced in the surface of the body and in the extremities than in the interior parts and organs.

This occlusion of the surface circulation can be easily observed and even measured by a simple test. Press the tip of the forefinger of one hand on the back of the other. A white spot will be formed where the blood has receded from the surface on account of the pressure. Now observe how quickly or how slowly the blood returns into this white patch.

Dr. Haig says that, if the reflux of the blood take place within two or three seconds, the circulation is normal and not obstructed by uric acid. If, however, the blood does not return for four or more seconds, it is a sign that the capillary circulation is obstructed by colloid uric acid occlusion.

In this connection I would call attention to the fact that the accumulation of carbonic acid in the cells and tissues, and the resulting oxygen starvation, may produce similar interference with the circulation and result in the same symptoms, including the slow reflux of blood after pressure, as those which Dr. Haig ascribes to the action of uric acid only.

When this obstruction of the circulation by uric or carbonic acid prevails throughout the body, the blood pressure is too high in the arterial blood vessels and in the interior organs, such as heart, lungs, brain, etc., and too low in the surface, the extremities and in the venous circulation. The return flow of the blood to the heart through the veins is sluggish and stagnant because the force from behind, that is, the arterial blood pressure, is obstructed by the uric acid which clogs the minute capillaries that form the connection between the arterial and the venous systems.

Because of this interference with the normal circulation and distribution of the blood, uric acid produces many annoying and deleterious effects. It irritates the nerves, the mucous membranes and other tissues of the body, thus causing headaches, rheumatic pains in joints and muscles, congestion of blood in the head, flushes, dizziness, depression, fainting and even epilepsy.

Other results of uric acid irritation are: inflammatory and catarrhal conditions of the bronchi, lungs, stomach, intestines, genitourinary organs; rapid pulse; palpitation of the heart; angina pectoris; etc.

These colloid substances occlude the minute excretory ducts in liver, spleen, kidneys and other organs, interfering with their normal functions and causing the retention of morbid matter in the system.

All these troublesome and destructive effects of uric acid poisoning may be greatly augmented by excessive accumulation of sulphuric, phosphoric and other acids, and by the formation of ptomaines and poisonous alkaloids during the metabolism of proteid substances.

The entire group of symptoms caused by the excess of uric acid in the system and the resulting occlusion of the capillary blood vessels by colloid substances is called *collemia* [a glutinous or viscid condition of the blood].

If in such a condition as collemia the amount of uric acid in the circulation is still farther increased by the taking of uric acid-producing food and drink and the saturation point of the blood is reached, that is, if the blood becomes overcharged with the acid, a curious phenomenon may be observed: **the collaemic symptoms suddenly disappear** as if by magic, giving way to a feeling of physical and mental buoyancy and strength.

This wonderful change has been wrought because the blood has lost its capacity for dissolving uric acid and holding it in solution and the acid has been precipitated, thrown out of the circulation and deposited in the tissues of the body.

After a period of rest, that is, when no uric acid- or xanthine-producing foods have been taken for some time, say, overnight, the blood regains its alkalinity and its capacity for dissolving and carrying uric acid and begins to reabsorb it from the tissues. As a consequence, the blood becomes again saturated with uric acid and the collaemic symptoms reappear.

This explains why the hilariousness and exaltation of spirits at the banquet is followed by "Katzenjammer" [hangover] in the morning. It also explains why many people do not feel fit for their day's work unless they take a stimulant of some kind on arising. Their blood is continually filled with uric acid to the point of saturation and the extra amount contained in the coffee or alcohol repeats the process of uric-acid precipitation, the temporary stimulation and relief.

Every time this precipitation of uric acid from the circulation is repeated, some of the morbid materials remain and accumulate in different parts and organs. If these irritating substances become lodged in the joints and muscles, arthritic or muscular rheumatism is the result. If acids, xanthines and oxalates of lime form earthy deposits along the walls of arteries and veins, these vessels harden and become inelastic, and their diameter is diminished. This obstructs the free circulation of the blood and causes malnutrition of the brain and other vital organs. Furthermore, the blood vessels become brittle and break easily and there is danger of hemorrhages.

This explains the origin and development of arteriosclerosis (hardening of the arteries) and apoplexy.

Apoplexy may also be caused by other acids and drug poisons which soften, corrode and destroy the walls of the blood vessels in the brain.

In individuals of different constitutions, accumulations of uric acid, xanthines, oxalates of calcium and various other earthy substances form stones, gravel or sandy deposits in the kidneys, the gall bladder and in other parts and organs.

The diseases caused by permanent deposits of uric acid in the tissues are called arthritic diseases, because the accumulations frequently occur in the joints.

Thus we distinguish two distinct stages of uric acid diseases: the **collaemic** stage, marked by an excess of uric acid in the circulation and resulting in occlusion of the capillary blood vessels, and the **arthritic** stage, marked by permanent deposits of uric acid and other earthy substances in the tissues of the body.

During the prevalence of the collaemic symptoms, that is, when the circulation is saturated with uric acid, the urine is also highly acid. When precipitation of the acid materials from the blood into the tissues has taken place, the amount of acid in the urine decreases materially.

I have repeatedly stated that xanthines have the same effect upon the system as uric acid. Caffeine and theobromine, the narcotic principles of coffee and tea, are xanthines; and so is the nicotine contained in tobacco. Peas, beans, lentils, mushrooms and peanuts, besides being very rich in uric acid-producing proteins, carry also large percentages of xanthines, which are chemically almost identical with uric acid and have a similar effect upon the organism and its functions.

From what has been said, it becomes clear why the meat-eater craves alcohol and xanthines. When by the taking of flesh foods the blood has become saturated with uric acid and the annoying symptoms of collaemia make their appearance in the forms of lassitude, headache and nervous depression, then alcohol and the xanthines contained in coffee, tea and tobacco will cause the precipitation of the acids from the circulation into the tissues of the body, and thus temporarily relieve the collaemic symptoms and create a feeling of well-being and stimulation.

Gradually, however, the blood regains its alkalinity and its acid-dissolving power and enough of the acid deposits are reabsorbed by the circulation to cause a return of the symptoms of collaemia. Then arises a craving for more alcohol, coffee, tea, nicotine or xanthine-producing foods in order to again obtain temporary relief and stimulation, and so on, ad infinitum.

The person addicted to the use of stimulants is never himself. His mental, moral and emotional equilibrium is always unbalanced. His brain is muddled with poisons and he lacks the self-control, the clear vision and steady hand necessary for the achievement of success in any line of endeavor.

We can now understand why one stimulant craves another, why it is almost impossible to give up one stimulant without giving up all others as well.

From the foregoing it will have become clear that **the stimulating effect of alcohol and of many so-called tonics depends upon their power to clear the circulation temporarily of uric and other acids.** Those who have read this chapter carefully, will know why this effect is deceptive and temporary and why it is followed by a return of the collaemic symptoms in aggravated form, and how these are gradually changed into chronic arthritic uric acid diseases.

In order to give a better idea of the various phases of uric acid poisoning, I have used the following illustration in some of my lectures:

A man may carry a burden of fifty pounds on his shoulders without difficulty or serious discomfort. Let this correspond to the normal solving-power and carrying-capacity of the blood for uric acid. Suppose you add gradually to the burden on the man's back until its weight has reached one-hundred and fifty pounds. He may still be able to carry the burden, but as the weight increases he will begin to show signs of distress. This increase of weight and the attendant discomfort correspond to the increase of uric acid in the blood and the accompanying symptoms of collaemia.

If you increase the burden on the man's shoulders still further, beyond his individual carrying-capacity, a point will be reached when he can no longer support its weight and will throw it off entirely. This climax corresponds to the saturation point of the blood, when the limit of its acid-carrying capacity is exceeded and its acid contents are precipitated into the tissues.

The Treatment of Acid Diseases

The treatment of acid diseases is the same as of all other diseases that are due to the violation of Nature's laws: purification of blood and tissues from within and building up of the vital fluids (blood and lymph) on a natural basis through normal habits of eating, dressing, bathing, breathing, working, resting and thinking as outlined in other parts of this volume.

In severe cases which have reached the chronic stage, the treatment must be supplemented by the more aggressive methods of strict diet, hydrotherapy, curative gymnastics, massage, manipulation and homeopathic medication.

Chapter XXVII

Fasting

Next in importance to building up the blood on a natural basis is the elimination of waste, morbid matter and poisons from the system. This depends to a large extent upon the right (natural) diet; but it must be promoted by the different methods of eliminative treatment: fasting, hydrotherapy, massage, physical exercise, air- and sunbaths and, in the way of medicinal treatment, by homeopathic, herb and vitochemical remedies.

Foremost among the methods of purification stands **fasting**, which of late years has become quite popular and is regarded by many people as a panacea for all human ailments. However, it is a two-edged sword. According to circumstances, it may do a great deal of good or a great deal of harm.

Kuhne, the German pioneer of Nature Cure, claimed that "disease is a unit," that it consists in the accumulation of waste and morbid matter in the system. Since his time, many "naturists" claim that fasting offers the best and quickest means for eliminating systemic poisons and other encumbrances.

To "fast it out" seems simple and plausible, but it does not always prove to be successful in practice. Fasting enthusiasts forget that the elimination of waste and morbid matter from the system is more of a chemical than a mechanical process. They also overlook the fact that **in many cases lowered vitality and weakened powers of resistance precede and make possible the accumulation of morbid matter in the organism.**

If the encumbrances consist merely of superfluous flesh and fat or of accumulated waste materials, fasting may be sufficient to break up the accumulations and to eliminate the impurities that are clogging blood and tissues.

If, however, the disease has its origin in other than mechanical causes, or if it is due to a weakened, negative constitution and lowered powers of resistance, fasting may aggravate the abnormal conditions instead of improving them.

We hear frequently of long fasts, extending over days and weeks, undertaken recklessly without the prescription and guidance of a competent medical adviser, without proper preparation of the system and the right subsequent treatment. Many a good constitution has thus been permanently injured and wrecked.

When Fasting Is Indicated

Persons of sanguine, vital temperament, with the animal qualities strongly developed, enslaved by bad habits and evil passions, will be greatly benefited by occasional short fasts. In such cases, the experience affords a fine drill in self-discipline, strengthening of self-control and conquest of the lower appetites.

Vigorous, fleshy people, positive physically and mentally, especially those who do not take sufficient physical exercise, should take frequent fasts of one, two, or three days' duration for the reduction of superfluous flesh and fat and for the elimination of systemic waste and other morbid materials. Such people should never eat more than two meals a day, and many get along best on one meal.

However, different temperaments and constitutions require different treatment and management. People of a nervous, emotional temperament, especially those who are below normal in weight and physically and mentally negative, may be seriously and permanently injured by fasting. They should never fast **except in acute diseases and during eliminative healing crises,** when Nature calls for the fast as a means of cure.

People of this type are usually thin, with weak and flabby muscles. Their vital activities are at a low ebb and their magnetic envelopes (aura) are wasted and attenuated like their physical bodies. The red aura, which is created by the action of the purely animal functions and forces, is more or less deficient or entirely lacking. Such people have the tendency to become abnormally sensitive to conditions in the magnetic field (the astral plane).

Next to the hypnotic or mediumistic process, there is nothing that induces abnormal psychism so quickly as fasting. During a prolonged fast, the purely animal functions of digestion, assimilation and elimination are almost completely at a standstill. This depression of the physical functions arouses and increases the psychic functions and may produce intense emotionalism and abnormal activity of the senses of the spiritual-material body, the individual thus becoming abnormally clairvoyant, clairaudient and otherwise sensitive to conditions on the spiritual planes of life.

This explains the spiritual exaltation and the visions of heavenly scenes and beings or the fights with demons which are frequently, indeed uniformly, reported by hermits, ascetics, saints, yogi, fakirs and dervishes.

Fasting facilitates hypnotic control of the sensitive by positive intelligences either on the physical or on the spiritual plane of being. In the one case we speak of hypnotism, in the other of mediumship, obsession or possession. These conditions are usually diagnosed by the regular practitioner as nervousness, nervous prostration, hysteria, paranoia, delusional insanity, double personality, mania, etc.

The destructive effects of fasting are intensified by solitude, grief, worry, introspection, religious exaltation or any other form of depressive or destructive mental and emotional activity.

Spirit controls often force their subjects to abstain from food, thus rendering them still more negative and submissive. Psychic patients, when controlled or obsessed, will frequently not eat unless they are forced or fed like an infant. When asked why they do not want to eat, these patients reply: "I mustn't. They will not let me." When we say: "Who?" the answer is: "These people. Don't you see them?" pointing to a void, and becoming impatient when told that no one is there. The regular school says delusion; we call it abnormal clairvoyance.

In other instances the control tells the subject that his food and drink are poisoned or unclean. To the obsessed victim these suggestions are absolute reality.

To place persons of the negative, sensitive type on prolonged fasts and thus to expose them to the dangers just described is little short of criminal. Such patients need an abundance of the most positive animal and vegetable foods in order to build up and strengthen their physical bodies and their magnetic envelopes, which form the dividing and protecting wall between the terrestrial plane and the magnetic field.

A **negative vegetarian diet,** consisting principally of fruits, nuts, cereal and pulses, but deficient in animal foods (the dairy products, eggs, honey) and in the vegetables growing in or near the ground **may result in conditions similar to those which accompany prolonged fasting.**

Animal foods are elaborated under the influence of a higher life-element[4] than that controlling the vegetable kingdom, and foods derived

---

4 This subject will be treated more fully in another volume of this series entitled "Natural Dietitics."

from the animal kingdom are necessary to develop and stimulate the positive qualities in man.

In the case of the psychic, who is already deficient in the physical (animal) and overdeveloped in the spiritual qualities, it is especially necessary, in order to restore and maintain the lost equilibrium, to build up in him the animal qualities.

How to Take an Occasional Therapeutic Fast

Before, during and after a therapeutic fast, everything must be done to keep elimination active, in order to prevent the reabsorption of the toxins that are being stirred up and liberated.

Fasting involves rapid breaking down of the tissues. This creates great quantities of worn-out cell materials and other morbid substances. Unless these poison-producing accumulations are promptly eliminated, they will be reabsorbed into the system and cause autointoxication.

To prevent this, bowels, kidneys and skin must be kept in active condition. The diet, for several days before and after the fast, should consist largely of uncooked fruits and vegetables and the different methods of natural stimulative treatment to assure proper bowel action should be systematically applied.

During a fast, every bit of vitality must be economized; therefore the passive treatments are to be preferred to active exercise, although a certain amount of exercise (especially walking) daily in the open air accompanied by deep breathing should not be neglected.

While fasting, intestinal evacuation usually ceases, especially where there is a natural tendency to sluggishness of the bowels. Injections [salt and baking soda enemas are best] are therefore in order and during prolonged fasts may be taken every few days.

By prolonged fasts we understand fasts that last from one to four weeks, short fasts being those of one, two or three days' duration.

Moderate drinking is beneficial during a fast as well as at other times; but excessive consumption of water, the so-called flushing of the system, is very injurious. Under ordinary conditions from five to eight glasses of water a day are probably sufficient; the quantity consumed must be regulated by the desire of the patient.

Those who are fasting should mix their drinking water with the juice of acid fruits, preferably lemon, orange or grapefruit. These juices act as eliminators and are fine natural antiseptics.

Never use distilled water, whether during a fast or at any

other time. Deprived of its own mineral constituents, distilled water leeches the mineral elements and organic salts out of the tissues of the body and thereby intensifies dysemic [blood deterioration] conditions.

While fasting, the right mental attitude is all-important. Unless you can do it with perfect equanimity, without fear or misgiving, do not fast at all. Destructive mental conditions may more than offset the beneficial effects of the fast.

To recapitulate: Never undertake a prolonged fast unless you have been properly prepared by natural diet and treatment, and never without the guidance of a competent Nature Cure doctor.

Fasting in Chronic Diseases

At all times some of our patients can be found fasting; but they do not begin until the right physiological and psychological moment has arrived, until the fast is indicated. When the organism, or rather the individual cell, is ready to begin the work of elimination, then assimilation should cease for the time being, because it interferes with the excretory processes going on in the system.

To fast before the system is ready for it, means mineral salts starvation and defective elimination.

Given a vigorous, positive constitution, encumbered with too much flesh and with a tendency to chronic constipation, rheumatism, gout, apoplexy and other diseases due to food poisoning, a fast may be indicated from the beginning. But it is different with persons of the weak, negative type.

Ordinarily, the organism resembles a huge sponge, which absorbs the elements of nutrition from the digestive tract. During a fast the process is reversed, the sponge is being squeezed and gives off the impurities contained in it.

However, this is a purely mechanical process and deals only with the mechanical aspect of disease: with the presence of waste matter in the system. It does not take into consideration the chemical aspect of disease. We have learned that most of the morbid matter in the system has its origin in the acid waste products of starchy and protein digestion.

In rheumatism and gout, the colloid (glue-like) and earthy deposits collect in the joints and muscular tissues; in arteriosclerosis, in the arteries and veins; in paralysis, epilepsy and kindred diseases, in brain and nerve tissues.

The accumulation of these waste products is due, in turn, to

a deficiency in the system of the alkaline, acid-binding and acid-eliminating mineral elements. In point of fact, almost every form of disease is characterized by a lack of these organic mineral salts in blood and tissues.

Stones, gravel (calculi), etc., grow in acid blood only, and must be dissolved and eliminated by rendering the blood alkaline. This is accomplished by the absorption of the alkaline salts, contained most abundantly in the juicy fruits, the leafy and juicy vegetables, the hulls of cereals and in milk.

How, then, are these all-important solvents and eliminators to be supplied to the organism by total abstinence from food?

Prolonged fasting undoubtedly lowers the patient's vitality and powers of resistance. But natural elimination of waste products and systemic poisons (healing crises) depends upon **increased** vitality and activity of the organism and the individual cells that compose it.

For these reasons we find, in most cases, that proper adjustment of the diet, both as to quality and quantity, together with the different forms of natural corrective and stimulative treatment, must precede the fasting.

The great majority of chronic patients have become chronics because their skin, kidneys, intestines and other organs of elimination are in a sluggish, atrophied condition. As a result, their system is overloaded with morbid matter.

Moreover, during the fast the system has to live on its own tissues, which are being broken down rapidly. This results in the production and liberation of additional large quantities of morbid matter and poisons, which must be eliminated promptly to prevent their reabsorption.

However, the atrophic condition of the organs of elimination makes this impossible and there are not enough alkaline mineral elements to neutralize the destructive acids. Therefore the impurities remain and accumulate in the system and may cause serious aggravations and complications.

Is it not wiser first of all to build up the blood on a normal basis by natural diet and to put the organs of elimination in good working order by the natural methods of treatment before fasting is enforced? This is, indeed, the **only rational** procedure and will always be followed by the best possible results.

When, under the influence of a rational diet, the blood has regained its normal composition, when mechanical obstructions to the free flow of blood and nerve currents have been removed by manipulative treatment, when skin, kidneys, bowels, nerves and nerve centers, in fact, every cell in the body has been stimulated into vigorous activity by the various methods of natural treatment, then the cells themselves begin to eliminate their morbid encumbrances. The waste materials are carried in the blood stream to the organs of elimination and incite them to acute reactions or healing crises in the form of diarrheas, catarrhal discharges, fevers, inflammations, skin eruptions, boils, abscesses, etc.

Now the sponge is being squeezed and cleansed of its impurities in a natural manner. The mucous membranes of stomach and bowels are called upon to assist in the work of housecleaning; hence the coated tongue, lack of appetite, digestive disturbances, nausea, biliousness, sour stomach, fermentation, flatulence and occasionally vomiting and purging.

These digestive disturbances are always accompanied by mental depression, the blues, homesickness, irritability, fear, hopelessness, etc.

With the advent of these cleansing and healing crises the physiological and psychological moment for fasting has arrived. All the processes of assimilation are at a standstill. The entire organism is eliminating.

We have learned that these healing crises usually arrive during the sixth week of natural treatment.

To take food now would mean to force assimilation and thereby to stop elimination and perchance to interfere with or to check a beneficial healing crisis.

Therefore we regard it as absolutely essential to stop eating as soon as any form of acute elimination makes its appearance and we do not give any food except acid fruit juices diluted with water until all signs of acute eliminative activity have subsided, whether this require a few days or a few weeks or a few months.

Some time ago I treated a severe case of typhoid malaria. No food, except water mixed with a little orange or lemon juice, passed the lips of the patient for eight weeks. When all disease symptoms had disappeared, we allowed a few days for the rebuilding of the intestinal mucous membranes. Thereafter food was administered with the usual precautions. The patient gained rapidly and within six weeks weighed more than before the fever. During the entire period I saw the patient only twice, the simple directions being carried out faithfully by his relatives.

Chapter XXVIII

Hydrotherapy Treatment of Chronic Disease

While in our treatment of acute diseases we use wet packs and cold ablutions to promote the radiation of heat and thereby to reduce the fever temperature, our aim in the treatment of **chronic** diseases is to arouse the system to acute eliminative effort. In other words, while in acute disease our hydropathic treatment is sedative, in chronic diseases it is stimulative.

The Good Effects of Cold-Water Applications

(1) Stimulation of the Circulation.

As before stated, cold water applied to the surface of the body arouses and stimulates the circulation all over the system. Blood counts before and after a cold-water application show a very marked increase in the number of red and white blood corpuscles. This does not mean that the cold water has in a moment created new blood cells, but it means that the blood has been stirred up and sent hurrying through the system, that the lazy blood cells which were lying inactively in the sluggish and stagnant blood stream and in the clogged and obstructed tissues are aroused to increased activity.

Undoubtedly, the invigorating and stimulating influence of cold sprays, ablutions, sitz baths, barefoot walking in the dewy grass or on wet stones and all other cold-water applications depends largely upon their electromagnetic effects upon the system. This has been explained in Chapter Ten, "Natural Treatment of Acute Diseases."

(2) Elimination of Impurities.

As the cold water drives the blood with increased force through the system, it flushes the capillaries in the tissues and cleanses them from the accumulations of morbid matter and poisons which are one of the primary causes of acute and chronic diseases.

As the blood rushes back to the surface it suffuses the skin, opens and relaxes the pores and the minute blood vessels or capillaries and thus unloads its impurities through the skin.

Why We Favor Cold Water

In the treatment of chronic diseases some advocates of natural methods of healing still favor warm or hot applications in the form of hot-water baths, different kinds of steam or sweat baths, electric light baths, hot compresses, fomentations, etc.

However, the great majority of Nature Cure practitioners in Germany have abandoned hot applications of any kind almost entirely because of their weakening and enervating aftereffects and because in many instances they have not only failed to produce the expected results, but aggravated the disease conditions.

We can explain the different effects of hot and cold water as well as of all other therapeutic agents upon the system by the Law of Action and Reaction. Applied to physics, this law reads: "Action and reaction are equal but opposite." I have adapted the Law of Action and Reaction to therapeutics in a somewhat circumscribed way as follows: "Every therapeutic agent affecting the human organism has a primary, **temporary,** and a secondary, **permanent** effect. The secondary, lasting effect is contrary to the primary, transient effect."

The first, temporary effect of warmth above the body temperature, whether it be applied in the form of hot air or water, steam or light, is to draw the blood into the surface. Immediately after such an application the skin will be red and hot.

The secondary and lasting effect, however (in accordance with the Law of Action and Reaction), is that the blood recedes into the interior of the body and leaves the skin in a bloodless and enervated condition subject to chills and predisposed to "catching cold."

On the other hand, the first, transient effect of cold-water applications upon the body as a whole or any particular part is to chill the surface and send the blood scurrying inward, leaving the skin in a chilled, bloodless condition. This lack of blood and sensation of cold are at once telegraphed over the afferent nerves to headquarters in the brain, and from there the command goes forth to the nerve centers regulating the circulation: "Send blood into the surface!"

As a result, the circulation is stirred up and accelerated throughout the system and the blood rushes with force into the depleted skin, flushing the surface of the body with warm, red blood and restoring to it the rosy color of health. **This is the secondary effect.** In other words, the well-applied cold-water treatment is followed by a good reaction and this is accompanied by many permanent beneficial results.

The drawing and eliminating primary effect of **hot** applications, of sweat baths, etc., is at best only **temporary,** lasting only a few minutes and is always followed by a weakening reaction, while the drawing and eliminating action of the **cold-water** applications, being the secondary, **lasting** effect, exerts an enduring, invigorating and tonic influence upon the skin which enables it to throw off morbid matter not merely for ten or fifteen minutes, as in the sweat bath under the infiuence of excessive heat, but continually, by day and night.

The Danger of Prolonged or Excessively Cold Applications

As we have pointed out in the chapter dealing with water treatment in acute diseases, only water at ordinary temperature, as it comes from well or faucet, should be used in hydropathic applications. It is positively dangerous to apply ice bags to an inflamed organ or to use icy water for packs and ablutions in febrile conditions.

Likewise, ice or icy water should not be used in the hydropathic treatment of chronic diseases. Excessive cold is as suppressive in its effects upon the organism as are poisonous antiseptics or antifever medicines.

The baths, sprays, douches, etc., should not be kept up too long. The duration of the cold-water applications must be regulated by the individual conditions of the patient and by his powers of reaction; but it should be borne in mind that it is the short, quick application that produces the stimulating, electromagnetic effects upon the system.

In the following pages are described some of the baths and other cold-water applications that are especially adapted to the treatment of chronic diseases.

How to Keep the Feet Warm

The proverb says: "Keep the head cool and the feet warm." This is good advice, but most people attempt to follow it by "doctoring" their cold feet with hot-water bottles, warming pans, hot bricks or irons, etc. These are excellent means of making the feet still colder, because "heat makes cold and cold makes heat."

In accordance with the Law of Action and Reaction, hot applications drive the blood away from the feet, while cold applications draw the blood to the feet. Therefore, if your feet are cold and bloodless (which means that the blood is congested in other parts of the body), walk barefoot in the dewy grass, in a cool brook, on wet stone pavements or on the snow.

Instead of putting a hot-water bottle to the feet of a bedridden invalid, bathe his feet with cold water, adding a little salt for its electric effect, then rub and knead (massage), and finish with a magnetic treatment by holding his feet between your hands and willing the blood to flow into them. This will have a lasting good effect not only upon the feet, but upon the entire organism.

The following cold-water applications are very effective for curing chronic cold feet:

(1) Foot Bath
Stand in cold water reaching up to the ankle for one minute only. Dry the feet with a coarse towel and rub them vigorously with the hands, or walk about briskly for a few minutes. Repeat if necessary.

(2) Leg Bath
a.   Stand in water up to the calves, then proceed as above.

b.   Stand in water up to the knees, then rub vigorously or walk as directed.

(3) Barefoot Walking
Walk barefoot in wet grass or on wet stone pavements several times a day, from ten to twenty minutes at a time, or less in case of weakness. The early morning dew upon the grass is especially beneficial; later in the day wet the grass or pavement with a hose. After barefoot walking, dry and rub the feet thoroughly and take a short, brisk walk in shoes and stockings.

(4) Indoor Water-Treading
Stand in a bathtub or large foottub containing about two inches of cold water, step and splash vigorously for several minutes, then dry and rub the feet and increase the circulation by walking around the room a few times.

(5) Foot Spray
Turn the full force of water from a hydrant or hose first on one foot, then on the other. Let the stream play alternately on the upper part of the feet and on the soles. The coldness and force of the water will draw the blood to the feet.

These applications are excellent as a means of stimulating and equalizing the circulation and a sure cure for cold and clammy feet, as well as for sweaty feet.

In this connection, we warn our readers most strongly against the use of drying powders or antiseptic washes to suppress foot-sweat. Epilepsy and other serious nervous disorders have been traced to this practice.

(6) Partial Ablutions

Partial ablutions with cold water are very useful in many instances, especially in local inflammation or where local congestion is to be relieved. The "Kalte Guss" [cold water splashing] forms an important feature of the Kneipp system of water cure.

Sprays or showers may be administered to the head, arms, chest, back, thighs, knees or wherever indicated, with a dipper, a sprinkler or a hose attached to the faucet or hydrant. The water should be of natural temperature and the "guss" of short duration.

(7) Limb Bath

Take up cold water in the hollow of the hands from a running faucet or a bucket filled with water, rub arms and legs briskly for a few minutes.

(8) Upper Body Bath

Stand in an empty tub, take water in the hollow of the hands from a running faucet or a bucket filled with cold water and rub briskly the upper half of the body from neck to hips, for two or three minutes. Use a towel or brush for those parts of the body that you cannot reach with the hands.

(9) Lower Body Bath

Proceed as in (8), rubbing the lower part of the body from the waist downward.

(10) Hip Bath

Sit in a large basin or in the bathtub in enough water to cover the hips completely, the legs resting on the door or against the sides of the tub. While taking the hip bath, knead and rub the abdomen.

Dry with a coarse towel, then rub and pat the skin with the hands for a few minutes.

The duration of the hip bath and the temperature of the water must be adapted to individual conditions. Until you are accustomed to cold water, use water as cool as can be borne without discomfort.

(11) The Morning Cold Rub

The essentials for a cold rub, and in fact for every cold-water treatment, are warmth of the body before the application, coolness of the water (natural temperature), rapidity of action and friction or exercise to stimulate the circulation. No cold-water treatment should be taken when the body is in a chilled condition.

Directly from the warmth of the bed, or after sunbath and exercise have produced a pleasant glow, go to the bathroom, sit in the empty tub with the stopper in place, turn on the cold water, and as it flows into the tub, catch it in the hollow of the hands and wash first the limbs, then the abdomen, then chest and back. Throw the water all over the body and rub the skin with the hands like you wash your face.

Do this quickly but thoroughly. The entire procedure need not take up more than a few minutes. By the time the bath is finished, there may be from two to four inches of water in the tub. Use a towel or brush for the back if you cannot reach it otherwise.

As long as there is a good reaction, the "cold rub" may be taken in an unheated bathroom even in cold weather.

After the bath, dry the body quickly with a coarse towel and finish by rubbing with the hands until the skin is dry and smooth and you are aglow with the exercise, or expose the wet body to the fresh air before an open window and rub with the hands until dry and warm.

A bath taken in this manner combines the beneficial effects of cold water, air, exercise and the magnetic friction of the hands on the body (life on life). No lifeless instrument or mechanical appliance can equal the dexterity, warmth and magnetism of the human hand.

The bath must be so conducted that it is followed by a feeling of warmth and comfort. Some persons will be benefited by additional exercise or, better still, a brisk walk in the open air, while others will get better results by returning to the warmth of the bed.

There is no better means for stimulating the general circulation and for increasing the eliminative activities of the system than this cold morning rub at the beginning of the day after the night's rest. If kept up regularly, its good effects will soon become apparent.

This method of taking a morning bath is to be preferred to the plunge into a tub filled with cold water. While persons with very strong constitutions may experience no ill effects, to those who are weak and do not react readily, the cold plunge might prove a severe shock and strain upon the system.

When a bathtub is not available, take the morning cold rub in the following manner:

Stand in an empty washtub. In front of you, in the tub, place a basin or bucket filled with cold water. Wet the hands or a towel and wash the body, part by part, from the feet upward, then dry and rub with the hands as directed.

(12) The Evening Sitz Bath

The morning cold rub is stimulating in its effects, the evening sitz bath is quieting and relaxing. The latter is therefore especially beneficial if taken just before going to bed.

The cold water draws the blood from brain and spinal cord and thereby insures better rest and sleep. It cools and relaxes the abdominal organs, sphincters, and orifices, stimulates gently and naturally the action of the bowels and of the urinary tract, and is equally effective in chronic constipation and in affections of the kidneys or bladder.

The sitz bath is best taken in the regular sitz bathtub made for the purpose, but an ordinary bathtub or a washtub or pan may be used with equally good effect.

Pour into the vessel a few inches of water at natural temperature, as it comes from the faucet, and sit in the water until a good reaction takes place—that is, until the first sensation of cold is followed by a feeling of warmth. This may take from a few seconds to a few minutes, according to the temperature of the water and the individual powers of reaction.

Dry with a coarse towel, rub and pat the skin with the hands, then, in order to establish good reaction, practice deep breathing for a few minutes, alternating with the internal massage described in a later chapter.

(13) The Head Bath

Loss or discoloration of the hair is generally due to the lack of hair-building elements in the blood or to sluggish circulation in the scalp and a diseased condition of the hair follicles. Nothing more effectually stimulates the flow of blood to brain and scalp or promotes the elimination of waste matter and poisons from these parts than the head bath together with scalp massage.

Under no circumstances use hair tonics, dandruff or eczema cures, or hair dyes. All such preparations contain poisons or at any rate strong antiseptics and germcides. Dandruff is a form of elimination and should not be suppressed. When the scalp is in good condition, it will disappear of its own accord.

The Diagnosis from the Eye reveals the fact that glycerine, quinine, resorcin and other poisonous antiseptics and stimulants absorbed from scalp cures and hair tonics and deposited in the brain are in many cases the real cause of chronic headaches, neuralgia, dizziness, roaring in the ears, loss of hearing and sight, mental depression, irritability and even insanity.

Cold water is an absolutely safe and at the same time a most effective means to promote the growth of hair, as many of our patients can testify.

Whenever you have occasion to wash the face, wash also the head thoroughly with cold water. While doing so, vigorously pinch, knead and massage the scalp with the finger tips. When feasible, turn the stream from a hydrant or a hose upon the head. This will add the good effect of friction to the coldness of the water.

Have your hair cut only during the third quarter of the moon. The ladies may clip off the ends of their hair during that period. Skeptics may smile at this as another evidence of ignorance and superstition. However, "fools deride,"etc. The country people in many parts of Europe, who are much closer and wiser observers of Nature and her ways than the conceited wise men of the schools, do their sowing and reaping in accordance with the phases of the moon. In order to insure vigorous growth, they sow and plant during the **growing** moon; but their cutting and reaping is done during the **waning** moon.

(14) The Eye Bath

For the eye bath the temperature of the water should be as cold as the sensitive eyeball can stand, but not cold enough to cause serious discomfort. A few grains of salt may be added to make the water slightly saline.

a. Submerge forehead and eyes in a basin of water, open and close the lids under water from six to eight times; repeat a few times.

b. Bend over a basin filled with water and with the hands dash the water into the open eyes.

c. Fill a glass eye-cup (which can be bought in any drug store or department store) with water, bend the head forward and press the cup securely against the eye; then bend backward and open and shut the lid a number of times.

Many ailments of the eyes, for instance, the much-dreaded cataract, are caused by defective circulation and the accumulation of impurities and poisons in the system in general and in the mechanism of the eyes in particular. All such cases yield readily to our combination of natural methods of treatment, such as water applications, massage and special exercises, combined with the general Nature Cure regimen.

In a large number of cases treated in our sanitarium, patients who had worn glasses for years were able to discard them. Weakened eyesight and many serious so-called incurable affections of the eye, including cataract and glaucoma, have been permanently cured.

Chapter XXIX

Air and Light Baths

Even among the adherents of Nature Cure there are those who think that air and light baths should be taken **out of doors** in warm weather only and in winter time only in well-heated rooms.

This is a mistake. The effect of the air bath upon the organism is subject to the same Law of Action and Reaction which governs the effects of water applications.

If the temperature of air or water is the same or nearly the same as that of the body, no reaction takes place, the conditions within the system remain the same. But if the temperature of air or water is considerably lower than the body temperature there will be a reaction.

In order to react against the chilling effect of cold air or water, the nerve centers which control the circulation send the blood to the surface in large quantities, flushing the skin with warm, red, arterial blood. The flow of the blood stream is greatly accelerated, and the elimination of morbid matter on the surface of the body is correspondingly increased.

What Is the Cause of Poor Skin Action?

Man is naturally an air animal. He breathes with the pores of the skin as well as with the lungs. However, the custom of hiding the body under dense, heavy clothing, thus excluding it from the life-giving influence of air and light, together with the habit of warm bathing, has weakened and enervated the skin of the average individual until it has lost its tonicity and is no longer capable of fulfilling its natural functions.

The compact, almost airtight layers of underwear and outer clothing made of cotton, wool, silk and leather prevent the ventilation of the skin and the escape of the morbid excretions of the body. The skin is an organ of absorption as well as of excretion; consequently the systemic poisons which are eliminated from the organism, if not removed by proper ventilation and bathing, are reabsorbed into the system just like the poisonous exhalations from the lungs are reinhaled and reabsorbed by people congregating in closed rooms or sleeping in unventilated bedrooms.

Who would think of keeping plants or animals continuously covered up, away from the air and light? We know they would wither and waste away, and die before long.

Nevertheless, civilized human beings have for ages hidden their bodies most carefully from sun and air, which are so necessary to their well-being. Is it any wonder that the human cuticle has become withered, enervated and atrophied, that it has lost the power to perform freely and efficiently its functions of elimination and absorption? Undoubtedly, this has much to do with the prevalence of disease.

In the iris of the eye the atrophied condition of the skin is indicated by a heavy, dark rim, the so-called scurf rim. It signifies that the skin has become anemic, the surface circulation sluggish and defective, and that the elimination of morbid matter and systemic poisons through the skin is handicapped and retarded. This, in turn, causes autointoxication and favors the development of all kinds of acute and chronic diseases.

The Importance of the Skin as an Organ of Elimination

Of late physiologists have claimed that the skin is not of great importance as an organ of elimination. Common experience and the Diagnosis from the Eye teach us differently. The black rim seen more or less distinctly in the outer rim of the iris in the eyes of the majority of people has been called the scurf rim, because it was found that this dark rim appears in the iris after the suppression of scurfy and other forms of skin eruptions and after the external or internal use of lotions, ointments and medicines containing mercury, zinc, iodine, arsenic or other poisons which suppress or destroy the life and activity of the skin.

Therefore, when we see in the iris of a person a heavy scurf rim, we can tell him at once: "Your cuticle is in a sluggish, atrophied condition, the surface circulation and elimination through the skin are not good and as a result of this there is a strong tendency to autointoxication, you take cold easily, and suffer from chronic catarrhal conditions." Therefore, a heavy scurf rim frequently indicates what is ordinarily called "a scrofulous condition."

This certainly shows the great importance of the skin as an organ of elimination and the necessity of keeping it in the best possible condition. It explains why an atrophied skin has so much to do with the causation of disease and why in the treatment of both acute and chronic ailments **air and cold water produce such wonderful results.**

The favorite method of diagnosis employed by Father Kneipp, the great water cure apostle, was to examine the skin of his patients. If the "jacket," as he called it, was in fairly good condition, he predicted a speedy recovery. If he found the "jacket" shriveled and dry, weakened and atrophied, he shook his head and informed the patient that it would take much time and patience to restore him to health. He, as well as other pioneers of the Nature Cure movement, realized that elimination is the keynote in the treatment of acute and chronic diseases.

When Air Baths Should Be Taken

On awakening in the morning and several times during the day, if circumstances permit, expose your nude body to the invigorating influence of the open air and the sunlight.

During the hot season of the year and in tropical countries the best time for taking air and sun baths is the early morning and the late afternoon.

Persons suffering from insomnia or nervousness in any form are in nearly every case greatly benefited by a short air bath taken just before retiring, either preceding or following the evening sitz bath, as may be most convenient.

Where Air Baths Should Be Taken

If at all possible, air baths should be taken out of doors. Every house should have facilities for air and sun baths, that is, an enclosure where the nude body can be exposed to the open air and the sunlight.

If the air bath out of doors is impracticable, it may be taken in front of an open window. But indoor air, even in a well-ventilated room, is more or less stagnant and vitiated, and at best only a poor substitute for the open air.

It is the breezy, moving outdoor air, permeated with sunlight and rich in oxygen and ozone, that generates the electric and magnetic currents which are so stimulating and vitalizing to everything that draws the breath of life.

This is being realized more and more, and air-bath facilities will in the near future be considered as indispensable in the modern, up-to-date house as is now the bathroom.

We predict that before many years the roofs of apartment houses will be utilized for this purpose and people will wonder how they ever got along without the air bath.

Our sanitarium has two large enclosures on its roof, open above and surrounded on all sides by wooden lattice work, which allows the air to circulate freely, but excludes observation from neighboring roofs and windows and the streets below. One compartment is for men and one for women, each provided with gymnastic apparatus and a separate spray room.

How Air Baths Should Be Taken

At first expose the nude body to cool air only for short periods at a time, until the skin becomes inured to it.

Likewise, unless you are well used to the sun, take air baths of short duration, say from ten to twenty minutes, until your skin and your nervous system have become accustomed to the influence of heat and strong light. Prolonged exposure to the glaring rays of the noonday sun might produce severe burning of the skin, aside from a possible harmful effect upon the nervous system.

The novice should protect head and eyes against the fierce rays of sunlight. This is best accomplished by means of a wide-brimmed straw hat of light weight. In cases where dizziness results from the effect of the heat upon the brain, a wet cloth may be swathed around the head or placed inside a straw hat.

It will be found very pleasurable and invigorating to take a cold shower or spray off and on during the sun bath and to allow the air to dry the body. This will also increase its electromagnetic effects upon the system.

The Friction Bath

While taking the air bath, the skin may be rubbed or brushed with a rough towel or a flesh brush in order to remove the excretions and the atrophied cuticle. The friction bath should always be followed by a spray or a cold-water rub.

At the time of the air bath, practice breathing exercises and the curative gymnastics appropriate to your condition. (See Chapters Twenty-Eight and Thirty on "Correct Breathing" and "Physical Exercise.")

If the air bath is taken at night, before retiring, the less active breathing exercises, as numbers 1, 3, 7 and 13, may be taken with good results, but all vigorous stimulating movements should be avoided.

As the plant prospers under the life-giving influence of water and light, so the cuticle of the human skin becomes alive and active under the natural stimulation of water, air and sunlight. From the foregoing paragraphs it will be seen why the air and light baths are regarded among the most important natural methods of treatment in all the great Nature Cure sanitariums of Germany.

.

Chapter XXX

Correct Breathing

The lungs are to the body what the bellows are to the fires of the forge. The more regularly and vigorously the air is forced through the bellows and through the lungs, the livelier burns the flame in the smithy and the fires of life in the body.

Practice deep, regular breathing systematically for one week, and you will be surprised at the results. You will feel like a different person, and your working capacity, both physically and mentally, will be immensely increased.

A plentiful supply of fresh air is more necessary than food and drink. We can live without food for weeks, without water for days, but without air only a few minutes.

The Process of Breathing

With every inhalation, air is sucked in through the windpipe or trachea, which terminates in two tubes called bronchi, one leading to the right lung, one to the left. The air is then distributed over the lungs through a network of minute tubes, to the air cells, which are separated by only a thin membrane from equally fine and minute blood vessels forming another network of tubes.

The oxygen contained in the inhaled air passes freely through these membranes, is absorbed by the blood, carried to the heart and thence through the arteries and their branches to the different organs and tissues of the body, fanning the fires of life into brighter flame all along its course and burning up the waste products and poisons that have accumulated during the vital processes of digestion, assimilation and elimination.

After the blood has unloaded its supply of oxygen, it takes up the carbonic acid gas which is produced during the oxidation and combustion of waste matter and carries it to the lungs, where the poisonous gases are transferred to the air cells and expelled with the exhaled breath. This return trip of the blood to the lungs is made through another set of blood vessels, the veins, and the blood, dark with the sewage of the system, is now called venous blood.

In the lungs the venous blood discharges its freight of

excrementitious poisons and gases, and by coming in contact with fresh air and a new supply of oxygen, it is again transformed into bright, red arterial blood, pregnant with oxygen and ozone, the life-sustaining elements of the atmosphere.

This explains why normal, deep, regular breathing is all-important to sustain life and as a means of cure. By proper breathing, which exercises and develops every part of the lungs, the capacity of the air cells is increased. This, as we have learned, means also an increased supply of life-sustaining and health-promoting oxygen to the tissues and organs of the body.

Bad Effects of Shallow Breathing

Very few people breathe correctly. Some, especially women, with tight skirtbands and corsets pressing on their vital organs, use only the upper part of their lungs. Others breathe only with the lower part and with the diaphragm, leaving the upper structures of the lungs inactive and collapsed.

In those parts of the lungs that are not used, slimy secretions accumulate, irritating the air cells and other tissues, which become inflamed and begin to decay. Thus a luxuriant soil is prepared for the tubercle bacillus, the pneumococcus and other disease-producing bacilli and germs.

This habit of shallow breathing, which does not allow the lungs to be thoroughly permeated with fresh air, accounts in a measure for the fact that one-third of all deaths result from diseases of the lungs. To one individual perishing from food starvation, thousands are dying from oxygen starvation.

Lung culture is more important than other branches of learning and training which require more time and a greater outlay of time, money and effort. In the Nature Cure regimen, breathing exercises play an important part.

Breathing Exercises

General Directions

The effectiveness of breathing exercises and of all other kinds of corrective movements depends upon the mental attitude during the time of practice. Each motion should be accompanied by the conscious effort to make it produce a certain result. Much more can be accomplished with mental concentration, by keeping your mind on what you are doing, than by performing the exercises in an aimless, indifferent way.

Keep in the open air as much as possible and at all events sleep with windows open.

If your occupation is sedentary, take all opportunities for walking out of doors that present themselves. While walking, breathe regularly and deeply, filling the lungs to their fullest capacity and also expelling as much air as possible at each exhalation. Undue strain should, of course, be avoided. This applies to all breathing exercises.

Do not breathe through the mouth. Nature intends that the outer air shall reach the lungs by way of the nose, whose membranes are lined with fine hairs in order to sift the air and to prevent foreign particles, dust and dirt, from irritating the mucous linings of the air tract and entering the delicate structures of the lungs. Also, the air is warmed before it reaches the lungs by its passage through the nose.

Let the exhalations take about double the time of the inhalations. This will be further explained in connection with rhythmical breathing.

Do not hold the breath between inhalations. Though frequently recommended by teachers of certain methods of breath culture, this practice is more harmful than beneficial.

The Proper Standing Position

Of great importance is the position assumed habitually by the body while standing and walking. Carelessness in this respect is not only unpleasant to the beholder, but its consequences are far-reaching in their effects upon health and the well-being of the organism.

On the other hand, a good carriage of the body aids in the development of muscles and tissues generally and in the proper functioning of cells and organs in particular. With the weight of the body thrown upon the balls of the feet and the center of gravity well focused, the abdominal organs will stay in place and there will be no strain upon the ligaments that support them.

In assuming the proper standing position, stand with your back to the wall, touching it with heels, buttocks, shoulders and head. Now bend the head backward and push the shoulders forward and away from the wall, still touching the wall with buttocks and heels. Straighten the head, keeping the shoulders in the forward position. Now walk away from the wall and endeavor to maintain this position while taking the breathing exercises and practicing the various arm movements.

Take this position as often as possible during the day and try to maintain it while you go about your different tasks that must be performed while standing. Gradually this position will become second nature, and you will assume and maintain it without effort.

When the body is in this position, the viscera are in their normal place. This aids the digestion materially and benefits indirectly the entire functional organism.

Persistent practice of the above will correct protruding abdomen and other defects due to faulty position and carriage of the body.

The following breathing exercises are intended especially to develop greater lung capacity and to assist in forming the habit of breathing properly at all times. The different movements should be repeated from three to six times, according to endurance and the amount of time at disposal.

1. With hands at sides or on hips, inhale and exhale slowly and deeply, bringing the entire respiratory apparatus into active play.

2. (To expand the chest and increase the air capacity of the lungs.)

   Jerk the shoulder **forward** in several separate movements, inhaling deeper at each forward jerk. Exhale slowly, bringing the shoulders back to the original position.

   Reverse the exercise, jerking the shoulders backward in similar manner while inhaling. Alternate the movements, forcing the shoulders first forward, then backward.

3. Stand erect, arms at sides. Inhale, raising the arms forward and upward until the palms touch above the head, at the same time raising on the toes as high as possible. Exhale, lowering the toes, bringing the hands downward in a wide circle until the palms touch the thighs.

4. Stand erect, hands on hips. Inhale slowly and deeply, raising the shoulders as high as possible, then, with a jerk, drop them as low as possible, letting the breath escape slowly.

5. Stand erect, hands at shoulders. Inhale, raising elbows sideways; exhale, bringing elbows down so as to strike the sides vigorously.

6. Inhale deeply, then exhale slowly, at the same time clapping the chest with the palms of the hands, covering the entire surface.

   (These six exercises are essential and sufficient. The following four may be practiced by those who are able to perform them and who have time and inclination to do so.)

7. Stand erect, hands at sides. Inhale slowly and deeply, at the same time bringing the hands, palms up, in front of the body

to the height of the shoulders. Exhale, at the same time turning the palms downward and bringing the hands down in an outward circle.

8. Stand erect, the right arm raised upward, the left crossed behind the back. Lean far back, then bend forward and touch the floor with the right hand, without bending the knees, as far in front of the body as possible. Raise the body to original posture, reverse position of arms, and repeat the exercise. Inhale while leaning backward and changing position of arms, exhale while bending forward.

9. Position erect, feet well apart, both arms raised. Lean back, inhaling, then bend forward, exhaling, touching the floor with both hands between the legs as far back as possible.

10. Horizontal position, supporting the body on palms and toes. Swing the right hand upward and backward, flinging the body to the left side, resting on the left hand and the left foot. Return to original position, repeat the exercise, flinging the body to the right side. Inhale while swinging backward, exhale while returning to position.

Diaphragmatic Breathing

The diaphragm is a large, flat muscle, resembling a saucer, which forms the division between the chest cavity and the abdominal cavity. By downward expansion it causes the lungs to expand likewise and to suck in the air. The pressure of air being greater on the outside of the body than within, it rushes in and fills the vacuum created by the descending diaphragm. As the diaphragm relaxes and becomes contracted to its original size and position, the air is expelled from the body.

11. (To stimulate the action of the diaphragm)

Lie flat on floor or mattress, the head unsupported. Relax the muscles all over the body, then inhale deeply with the diaphragm only, raising the wall of the abdomen just below the ribs without elevating either the chest or the lower abdomen. Take about four seconds to inhale, then exhale in twice that length of time, contracting the abdomen below the ribs.

12. (Internal massage)

Lie on your back on a bed or couch, knees raised. Relax thoroughly, exhale and hold the breath after exhalation. While doing so, push the abdomen out and draw it in as far as possible each way. Repeat these movements as long as you can hold the breath without straining, then breathe deeply and regularly for several minutes, then repeat the massage movements.

Next to deep breathing, I consider this practice of greater value than any other physical exercise. It imparts to the intestines an other abdominal organs a "washboard" motion which acts as a powerful stimulant to all the organs in the abdominal cavity. Internal massage is especially beneficial in chronic constipation. This exercise may be performed also while standing or walking. It should be practiced two or three times daily.

Breathing Exercises to Be Taken in Bed

13. With hands at side, inhale slowly and deeply, as directed in Exercise Number (1), filling and emptying the lungs as much as possible, but without straining. Practice first lying on the back, then on each side.

14. Using one- or two-pound dumbbells, position recumbent on back, arms extended sideways, dumbbells in hands. Raise the arms with elbows rigid, cross arms over the chest as far as possible, at the same time expelling the air from the lungs. Extend the arms to the sides, inhaling deeply and raising the chest.

15. Lie flat on the back, arms at sides. Grasping the dumbbells, extend the arms backward over the head, inhaling. Leave them in this position for a few seconds, then raise them straight above the chest, and lower them slowly to the original position. Exhale during the second half of this exercise.

As a variation, cross the arms in front of the body instead of bringing to sides.

Rhythmical Breathing

It is a fact not generally known to us western people (our attention had to be called to it by the "Wise Men of the East"), that in normal, rhythmical breathing exhalation and inhalation take place through one nostril at a time: for about one hour through the right nostril and then for a like period through the left nostril.

The breath entering through the right nostril creates **positive** electro-magnetic currents, which pass down the right side of the spine, while the breath entering through the left nostril sends **negative** electro-magnetic currents down the left side of the spine. These currents are transmitted by way of the nerve centers or ganglia of the sympathetic nervous system, which is situated alongside the spinal column, to all parts of the body.

In the normal, rhythmical breath exhalation takes about twice the time of inhalation. For instance, if inhalation require four seconds, exhalation, including a slight natural pause before the new inhalation, requires eight seconds.

The balancing of the electro-magnetic energies in the system depends to a large extent upon this rhythmical breathing, hence the importance of deep, unobstructed, rhythmic exhalation and inhalation.

In order to establish the natural rhythm of the breath when it has been impaired through catarrhal affections, wrong habits of breathing, or other causes, the following exercise, practiced not less than three times a day (preferably in the morning upon arising, at noon, and at night), will prove very beneficial in promoting normal breathing and creating the right balance between the positive and the negative electro-magnetic energies in the organism.

The Alternate Breath

Exhale thoroughly, then close the right nostril and **inhale through the left.** After a slight pause change the position of the fingers and **expel the breath slowly through the right nostril.** Now **inhale** through the **right** nostril and, reversing the pressure upon the nostrils, **exhale** through the **left.**

Repeat this exercise from five to ten times, always allowing twice as much time for exhalation as for inhalation. That is, count three, or four, or six for inhalation and six, eight, or twelve, respectively, for exhalation, according to your lung capacity. **Let your breaths be as deep and long as possible, but avoid all strain.**

This exercise should always be performed before an open window or, better yet, in the open air, and the body should not be constricted and hampered by tight or heavy clothing.

Alternate breathing may be practiced standing, sitting, or in the recumbent position. The spine should at all times be held straight and free, so that the flow of the electro-magnetic currents be not obstructed. If taken at night before going to sleep, the effect of this exercise will be to induce calm, restful sleep.

While practicing the "alternate breath," fix your attention and concentrate your power of will upon what you axe trying to accomplish. As you inhale through the right nostril, will the magnetic currents to flow along the right side of the spine, and as you inhale through the left nostril, consciously direct the currents to the left side.

There is more virtue in this exercise than one would expect, considering its simplicity. It has been in practice among the Yogi of India since time immemorial.

The wise men of India knew that with the breath they absorbed not only the physical elements of the air, but life itself. They taught that this primary force of all forces, from which all energy is derived, ebbs and flows in rhythmical breath through the created universe. Every living thing is alive by virtue of and by partaking of this cosmic breath.

The more positive the demand, the greater the supply. Therefore, while breathing deeply and rhythmically in harmony with the universal breath, **will** to open yourself more fully to the inflow of the life force from the source of all life in the innermost parts of your being.

This intimate connection of the individual soul with the great reservoir of life must exist. Without it life would be an impossibility.

Warning

While the alternate breathing exercises are very valuable for overcoming obstructions in the air passages, for establishing the habit of rhythmic breathing and for refining and accelerating the vibratory activities on the physical and spiritual planes of being, they must be practiced with great caution. These, and other "Yogi" breathing exercises, are powerful means for developing abnormal psychical conditions. They are therefore especially dangerous to those who are already inclined to be physically and mentally negative and sensitive. Such persons must avoid all practices which tend to refine excessively the physical body and to develop prematurely and abnormally the sensory organs of the spiritual body. The most dangerous of these methods are long extended fasting, raw food diet, that, is, a diet consisting of fruits, nuts, oils and raw vegetables and excluding the dalry products, "Yogi" breathing, and "sitting in the silence." That is, sitting in darkness, in seclusion or in company with others, while keeping the mind in a passive, receptive condition for extraneous impressions. These practices tend to develop very dangerous phases of abnormal and subjective psychism, such as clairvoyance, clairaudience, mediumship and obsession.

Chapter XXXI

Physical Exercise

Aside from breathing, gymnastics in general—or in the case of illness or deformity, special corrective and curative exercises—should be taken every day.

Physical exercise has similar effects upon the system as hydrotherapy, massage and manipulative treatment. It **stirs up the morbid accumulations in the tissues, stimulates the arterial and venous circulation, expands the lungs to their fullest capacity,** thereby increasing the intake of oxygen, and most effectively **promotes the elimination of waste and morbid materials** through skin, kidneys, bowels and the respiratory tract.

Furthermore, well-adapted, systematic physical exercises tend to correct dislocations of spinal vertebrae and other bony structures. They relax and soften contracted and hardened muscles and ligaments and tone up those tissues which are weakened and abnormally relaxed. Regular physical exercise means increased blood supply, improved nutrition and better drainage for all the vital organs of the body.

By means of systematic exercise, combined with deep breathing, the liberation and distribution of electromagnetic energies in the system are also greatly promoted.

Most persons who have to work hard physically are under the impression that they need not take special exercises. This, however, is a mistake. In nearly all kinds of physical labor only certain parts of the body are called into action and only certain sets of muscles exercised, while others remain inactive. **This favors unequal development,** which is injurious to the organism as a whole. It is most necessary that the ill effects of such one-sided activity be counteracted by exercises and movements that bring into active play all the different parts of the body, especially those that are neglected during the hours of work.

Systematic physical exercise is an absolute necessity for brain workers and those following sedentary occupations. They not only need breathing gymnastics and corrective movements mornings and evenings, but should take regular daily walks, no matter what the condition of the weather. Unless they do this faithfully, their circulation will become sluggish and their organs of elimination inactive. The cells and tissues of their bodies will gradually become clogged with morbid encumbrances, and this will inevitably lead to physical and mental deterioration.

General Rules

a. Weak persons and those suffering from malignant diseases, such as cancer, tuberculosis, heart trouble, asthma, or from displacements and ruptures, or who are liable to apoplectic seizures, etc., should not take these or any other vigorous exercises except under the supervision of a competent physician.

b. At least twice a day all parts of the respiratory apparatus should be thoroughly exercised (see Chapter Twenty-Eight on Breathing Exercises). Deep breathing should accompany every corrective movement, whether it be a special breathing exercise or not.

c. Begin your exercises each day with light movements and change gradually to more vigorous ones, then reverse the process, ending with light, relaxing movements.

d. When beginning to take systematic exercise, do not make the separate movements too vigorous or continue them too long. If any of them cause pain or considerable strain, omit them until the body becomes stronger and more flexible. The muscular soreness often resulting from exercise at the beginning is, as a rule, of little consequence and disappears before long. The different movements should be practiced in spite of it, because that is the only way to relieve and overcome this condition.

e. Stop when you begin to feel tired. Never overdo; you should feel refreshed and relaxed after exercising, not tired and shaky.

f. Do not take vigorous exercise of any kind within an hour and a half after eating, nor immediately before meals. It is a good plan to rest and relax thoroughly for about fifteen minutes before sitting down to the table.

g. Whenever practicable, exercise out of doors. If indoors, perform the movements near an open window or where there is a current of fresh air.

h. Exercise undressed, if possible, or in a regular gymnasium suit that gives free play to all the muscles. If dressed, loosen all tight clothing. Ladies should wear their garments suspended from the shoulders by means of shoulder braces, or so-called reform waists, the skirts being fastened to these.

i. Always relax physically and mentally before taking exercise.

j. Apparatus is not necessary to produce results. However, dumbbells, wands or Indian clubs may be used, but they should not be too heavy. One-pound dumbbells are sufficiently heavy in most cases. The exercises described here are intended for muscular control, flexibility, improvement of the circulation and increased activity of the vital functions rather than for mere animal strength.

In the following paragraphs we offer a selection of corrective movements, graduated from the more simple to those requiring considerable agility and effort.

In practicing these exercises, it is best to alternate them, that is, to select, say, six or seven movements, suited to individual conditions with a view to secure all-around general development and special practice for those parts and organs of the body that need extra attention. The time at your disposal will also have to be considered.

Practice these exercises daily for a week. For the following week select six different exercises, then six more for the third week, and so on, supplementing the list here given as may be required by your particular needs. Then start over again in a similar manner.

This is better than doing the same stunts every day. It promotes all-around development of the body and keeps the interest from flagging.

Corrective Gymnastics

1. Raise the arms forward (at the same time beginning to inhale), upward above the head, and backward as far as possible, bending back the head and inhaling deeply. Now exhale slowly, at the same time lowering arms and head and bending the body downward until the fingers touch the toes. **Keep the knees straight.** Inhale again, raising arms upward and backward as before. Repeat from six to ten times.

   For exercising the muscles between the ribs and the abdominal muscles in the back:

2. Inhale slowly and deeply, with arms at side. Now exhale, and at the same time bend to the left as far as possible, raising the right arm straight above the head and **keeping the left arm close to the side of the body.** Assume the original position with a quick movement, at the same time inhaling. Exhale as before, bending to the right and raising the left arm. Repeat a number of times.

   For making the chest flexible. Also excellent for the digestive organs:

3. **Chest Stretcher:** This exercise must be performed vigorously, the movements following one another in rapid succession:

   Stand erect. Throw the arms backward so that the palms

touch (striving to bring them higher with each repetition), at the same time rising on the toes and inhaling. Without pausing, throw the arms forward and across the chest, the **right** arm uppermost, striking the back with both hands on opposite sides, at the same time exhaling and lowering the toes. Throw the arms back immediately, touching palms, rising on toes and inhaling as before, then bring them forward and across the chest again, **left** arm upper most. Repeat from ten to twenty times.

An excellent massage and vibratory movement for the lungs.

4. Exercises for filling out scrawny necks and hollow chests:

Stand erect. Without raising or lowering the chin and **without bending the neck,** push the head forward as far as possible, then relax. Repeat a number of times. Push the head straight back in similar manner, making an effort to push it farther back each time. Do not bend the neck. Repeat.

Stand erect. Bend the head toward the right shoulder as far as possible, then relax. **Do not rotate the head.** Repeat.

Bend the head to the left shoulder in a similar manner, then alternate the two movements.

Stand erect. Bend the head **forward** as far as possible, making an effort to bring it down farther each time. Relax.

Bend the head **backward** as far as possible.

Bend the head first forward, then backward. Repeat.

5. For exercising the muscles of the chest and the upper arm.

Stand erect, elbows to sides, hands closed on chest, thumbs inward. Thrust out the arms vigorously and quickly, first straight ahead, then to the sides, then straight up, then straight downward, then backward. Repeat each movement a number of times, then alternate them, each time bringing arms back and hands to the original position quickly and forcefully.

As a variation, raise the elbows sideways to shoulder height with fists on shoulders, then strike vigorously as before, opening the palms and stretching the fingers with each thrust. Repeat from ten to twenty times or until tired.

6. Stand erect, hands on hips. Keeping the legs straight, rotate the trunk upon the hips, bending first forward, then to the right, then backward, then to the left. Repeat a number of times, then rotate in the opposite direction.

Especially valuable to stir up a sluggish liver:

7. Lie flat on your back on a bed or, better still, a mat on the

floor, hands under head. Without bending knees, raise the right leg as high as possible and lower it slowly. Repeat a number of times, then raise the other leg, then alternate. As the abdomen becomes stronger, raise both legs at once, keeping knees straight. **It is important that the legs be lowered slowly.**

For exercising the abdominal muscles and strengthening the pelvic organs. This and the following exercise are especially valuable for remedying female troubles:

8. Lie flat on back, arms folded on chest. Place the feet under a chair or bed to keep them in position. Raise the body to a sitting posture, keeping knees, back and neck straight. Lower the body **slowly** to its original position. Repeat from five to ten times, according to strength.

Supplementary Exercises

9. **Stride-stand** position (feet about one-half yard apart). Raise the arms sideways until even with the shoulders, then, without bending the back, rotate the trunk upon the hips, first to the right, then to the left.

   As a variation of this exercise, rotate from the waist only, keeping the hips motionless.

   An excellent massage for the internal organs:

10. See-saw motion:

    Stride-stand position, arms raised sideways. Bend to the right until the hand touches the floor, left arm raised high. Resume original position. Repeat several times, then bend to the left side, then alternate.

11. Chopping exercise:

    Stride-stand position. Clasp the hands above the left shoulder. Swing the arms downward and between the legs, bending well forward. Return to position and repeat a number of times, then repeat with hands on right shoulder, then alternate.

12. Cradle rock:

    Clasp hands over head, elbows straight. Bend the trunk to the right and left side alternately and without pausing a number of times.

13. Stand erect, feet together. Jump to the stride-stand position, at the same time raising arms sideways to shoulders, jump back to original position and lower arms. Repeat from ten to twenty times.

14. Lie flat on back, arms at side, legs straight. Raise both legs

till they are at right angles with body. From this position sway legs to the right and left side alternately.

15. Lie flat on back, arms extended over head. Swing arms and legs upward simultaneously, touching the toes with the hands in midair, balancing the body on the hip bones and lower part of spine. Return to original position and repeat.

This is a difficult and strenuous exercise, and should not be attempted at first:

16. Lie flat on stomach, hands under shoulders, palms downward, fingers turned inward, about six inches apart. This will give free play to the muscles of the chest. Raise the upper half of the body on the hands and arms as high as possible, keeping the body straight. Return to position and repeat until slightly fatigued.

17. Same position as before. Raise the entire body on hands and toes, keeping arms and legs straight. Return to relaxed position and repeat the exercise.

As a variation, sway forward and backward while in the raised position.

18. Lie flat on stomach, arms extended in front. Fling the arms upward and raise the upper part of the body as high as possible, **keeping the legs straight.** Return to position and repeat, but avoid excessive strain.

19. Same position as before, but hands on hips or clasped in back. Raise upper part of body without assistance from hands or arms.

20. Rocking chair motion:

Sit on a mat or bed, legs straight, arms at side. Recline so that the upper part of the body almost touches the mat, at the same time swinging the legs upward. Return to original position and repeat without any pause between the movements, rocking back and forth until slightly tired.

As you get stronger, clasp the hands behind the head. As a variation, rock with the knees bent, hands clasped below them.

Special Exercises for Reducing Flesh and Strengthening the Abdominal Organs

21. Lie flat on stomach, heels and toes together, hands stretched out in front. Fling head and arms upward, at the same time raising the legs, knees straight. **Avoid straining.**

22. Same position, hands clasped on back, feet together. Roll from side to side.

23. Lie flat on back, seize a bar (bed rail or rung of chair) just behind the head. Keeping the feet close together, raise the legs **as high as possible,** then swing them from side to side. As a variation, swing legs in a circle without flexing the knees.

24. Same position. Raise and lower the legs up and down without letting them touch the floor, keeping the knees straight.

25. Lie flat on the back, fold the hands loosely across the stomach. Raise and lower the upper body without quite touching the floor.

26. Stand erect, heels together, arms raised above the head. Bend forward and downward, endeavoring to place the palms of the hands on the floor in front of the body without flexing the knees. Return slowly to original position and repeat.

27. Stand erect, hands on hips. Keeping the body motionless from the hips downward, sway the upper part of the body from side to side and forward and backward, and in a circle to right and left.

28. Stand erect, raise the arms above the head. Rotate the trunk upon the hips with extended arms, bending as far as possible in each direction, but avoiding undue strain. These are strenuous movements and should not be carried to excess or performed very long at a time.

Physical Exercises for Invalids

Persons who are very weak and unable to be on their feet for any length of time need not, for this reason, forego the benefits to be derived from systematic physical exercise.

A low chair, with straight or very lightly curved back and no arms, or a rocking chair of similar construction with a wedge placed under the rockers in such a manner as to keep the chair steady at a suitable angle, is well adapted to the practice of a number of corrective movements, such as rotating of hips and waist, forward and sideward bending of the trunk, the various arm and neck exercises, bending and twisting of feet and toes, the internal massage (Exercise Number 12) and "Breathing Exercises to be Taken in Bed," in previous Chapter.

Chapter XXXII

Manipulative Treatment

Massage

Massage has very much the same effects upon the system as the cold-water treatment. It accelerates the circulation, draws the blood into the surface, relaxes and opens the pores of the skin, promotes the elimination of morbid matter and increases and stimulates the electromagnetic energies in the body.

We have learned that one of the primary causes of chronic disease is the accumulation of waste matter and systemic poisons in the tissues of the body. These morbid encumbrances clog the capillaries, thus obstructing the circulation and interfering with or preventing the normal activity of the organs of elimination, especially the skin.

The deep-going massage, the squeezing, kneading, rolling and stroking, actually **squeezes the stagnant blood and the morbid accumulations out of the tissues** into the venous circulation, speeds the venous blood, charged with waste products and poisons, on its way to the lungs and enables the arterial blood with its freight of oxygen and nourishing elements to flow more freely into the less-obstructed tissues and organs.

Through manipulation of the fleshy tissues, the blood is drawn to the surface of the body and in that way the elimination of morbid matter through the relaxed and opened pores of the skin is greatly facilitated.

Very important are the electromagnetic effects of good massage upon the system. The positive magnetism of the operator will stir up and intensify the latent electromagnetic energies in the body of the patient, very much like a piece of iron or steel is magnetized by rubbing it with a horseshoe magnet. The more normal and positive, morally and mentally as well as physically, the operator, the more marked will be the good effects of the treatment upon the weak and negative patient.

Magnetic Treatment

The beneficial effect of magnetic treatment is not so much due to the actual transmission of vital force from operator to patient as to the arousing and stimulating of the latent, inactive electromagnetic energies of the latter, the polarizing of his magnetic forces.

The horseshoe magnet does not impart its own magnetism to the piece of iron which is rubbed with it, but the electromagnetic energies in the magnet arouse to vibratory activity the latent electromagnetic energies in the iron. This is proved by the fact that both magnet and iron will remain magnetic as long as they are used for magnetizing other substances, but through disuse both will lose their magnetic qualities.

I am often asked by my operators and others: "How can I best develop my magnetism?" and "Is there danger of losing my vitality and becoming 'negative' by treating the sick in this way?" It is true that manipulative work, like everything else, can be overdone and produce harmful effects upon the operator. But within reasonable limits, massage and magnetic treatments will not deplete the person giving them, providing he keeps his system in good condition. His own vibrations must be harmonious on all planes of being, the physical, mental, moral and spiritual. He must be inspired and actuated by the **faith that he CAN heal,** by the **positive will to heal,** and by sympathy for the one he is trying to benefit.

Such an operator makes himself the instrument for the transmission of life force, which is healing force, from the Source of all life. "As he gives, so he receives"; for this is the basic law of the universe, the Law of Compensation. If he gives the treatments in the right spirit, **he will gain vital force instead of losing it.** He will actually **feel** his own intensified life vibrations and after treating he will experience a feeling of buoyancy and elation which nothing else can impart to him. "He who loses his life shall find it."

Like a musician who tunes up (puts in harmonious vibration) the relaxed strings of his instrument, so the magnetic healer tunes up and harmonizes the weakened and discordant vibrations of his patient.

Good massage will produce electromagnetic effects even though the operator is not aware of it and does not understand the underlying laws; but his work will gain in power and effectiveness in direct proportion to the conscious efforts he makes to benefit his patients by the influence of these higher and finer forces.

I have frequently noticed in my own manipulative work how much the conscious and concentrated effort of the will has to do with its effectiveness. Often, when I had given the usual massage or osteopathic treatment and the patient still complained of pain in a certain locality of the body, I would lay my hands on the affected area and **concentrate my will** upon dissolving the congestion in that particular part or organ and upon harmonizing its discordant vibrations. Very shortly, usually within a few minutes, the congestion would be relieved and the pain would subside.

The electromagnetic energies of the organism can be controlled by the will and either concentrated to or sent away from any part of the body, just as the circulation of the blood can be controlled. The latter I saw done by a hypnotist who made the blood flow into and out of the arms and hands of one of his subjects simply by the power of his will.

While this was accomplished by means of a destructive process, it taught me a most valuable lesson regarding the power of the will to control physical conditions.

Try it yourself. Next time when you have one of your annoying headaches, recline comfortably in a chair or on a couch, relax completely and then **Will the blood to flow away from the brain** in order to relieve the congestion and the attendant pain. Many of my patients have learned to treat themselves successfully in this way.

It is obvious that magnetic treatment will not remove pain permanently if the latter is due to irritation caused by a subluxated bone or by some foreign body or by local accumulation of morbid matter and poisons in any part or organ. In all such cases the local cause of the irritation must be removed before the pain can subside or disappear.

Spinal Manipulation and Adjustment: History

In many European countries "bonesetters" have, in a crude way, been treating strains and sprains of the spinal column since time immemorial. These bonesetters usually belong to the peasantry and the art has been transmitted in the same families from father to son for many generations.

Incidentally, these simple people observed that their treatment relieved not only sprained, tired and painful backs—the result primarily aimed at—but frequently exerted a favorable influence upon disease processes in remote organs and parts. This empirical discovery has gradually led to a wider application of this method of treatment.

The various modern systems of spinal manipulation, namely, osteopathy, chiropractic, naprapathy, neuropathy, spondylotherapy and our own neurotherapy, are all of distinctly American origin.

During the last quarter century millions of Americans through personal experience have become staunch adherents to one or more of these systems of treatment. This fact has been instrumental in directing the attention of numerous sincere and scientific investigators to the spinal column with its associated structures as a mechanism through which to apply therapeutic measures. It therefore behooves every health seeker to acquaint himself with the theories and claims of these various systems of manipulative treatment.

Osteopathy

The autobiography of Dr. A. T. Still contains the following interesting statement:

> "In the year 1874 I proclaimed that a disturbed artery marked the beginning to an hour and a minute when disease began to sow its seeds of destruction in the human body. That in no case could it be done without a broken or suspended current of arterial blood, which by Nature was intended to supply and nourish all nerves, ligaments, muscles, skin, bones and the artery itself. . . . The rule of the artery must be absolute, universal and unobstructed or disease will be the result. I proclaimed then and there that all nerves depend wholly on the arterial system for their qualities such as sensation, nutrition and motion, even though by the law of reciprocity they furnish force, nutrition and motion to the artery itself."

It may be argued that as early as 1805 the Ling System of Swedish Movement was founded on the same principle, namely, "permanent health through perfect circulation." The evidence at hand, however, strongly suggests that the founder of osteopathy arrived at his conclusions independently.

The further claims of Dr. Still as to the cause and cure of disease are briefly as follows: Partial displacements of any of the various bones of the body exert pressure on neighboring **blood vessels,** thereby interfering with the circulation to the corresponding organs. These displacements, called "bony lesions," are best "reduced" by manipulations called osteopathic "moves."

Chiropractic

In 1895, Dr. D. D. Palmer put forth the following claims as to the cause and cure of diseases: Sprains of the spine result in partial displacement of one or more of the vertebrae which go to make up the spinal column, thus exerting pressure on the neighboring nerves. This shuts off the vitality of the organs supplied by the affected nerves, hence disease results. These displacements, called "vertebral subluxations," are best "adjusted" by means of manipulations in the form of chiropractic "thrusts."

As soon as osteopathy and chiropractic were properly established, the more broad-minded exponents of both systems began mutual investigation and amalgamation. As a result, we find that only seven years after the birth of chiropractic, osteopathic literature began to mention vertebral subluxations as pressing on **nerves,** thereby causing disease. On the other hand, advanced chiropractors soon began to realize the importance of relaxing tense muscles prior to delivering their thrusts. They also began to pay attention to the bony lesions other than those occurring in the spine. Many of the chiropractic principles and much of its technique of today has been gleaned from osteopathy, while the reverse statement holds equally true.

Naprapathy

The "connective tissue doctrine of disease" was first proclaimed by Dr. Oakley Smith in 1907. It may be briefly stated as follows: A vertebra does not become misplaced without being fractured or completely dislocated. What is called a bony lesion by the osteopath and a subluxation by the chiropractor, is in reality a "ligatight," that is, a shrunken condition of the connective tissue forming the various ligaments that bind the vertebrae together.

Ligatights are best "corrected" by means of naprapathic "directos." These differ from chiropractic thrusts in that they aim not at adjusting subluxated vertebrae but at stretching definite strands of shrunken connective tissue. Ligatights occur not only in the spine but also in other parts of the body.

Neuropathy

This system of manipulative treatment was originated in 1899 by Drs. John Arnold and Harry Walter of Philadelphia. Their claims may be briefly stated as follows: Morbid matter, poisons and irritants of various kinds, acting upon the vasomotor nerves which control the blood vessels, produce abnormal changes in circulation which, if perpetuated, finally lead to disease manifestations. The nerve impulses coming from diseased parts travel to the spinal cord and, like all other nerve impulses, are transmitted along those branches of the spinal nerves which supply the structures (muscles, blood vessels, etc.) along each side of the spine. Here these impulses bring about abnormal circulatory changes similar to those found in the diseased organs or parts.

Since nerve impulses are transmitted from diseased organs to the spine, it is evident that they can be made to travel also in the reverse direction. Neuropathic treatment, therefore, consists of manipulations and thermal applications which aim at correcting the abnormal circulatory changes as found in the spine, thereby correcting corresponding abnormal processes in the organs or parts supplied by the nerves coming from that region of the spine.

These men also emphasized the fact that the circulation within the blood vessels, being propelled by the heart, needs less attention during disease than the circulation of the fluids in the spaces between the cells and through the lymph vessels and glands. Neuropathy, therefore, also lays great stress on applying manipulation and thermal applications to the lymphatic system.

Neurotherapy

While the exponents of the above systems of spinal manipulation differ widely in their theories as to the cause of disease and the means of removing such cause, their methods of treatment furnish considerable evidence of satisfactory results. This seems to suggest that there must be some real value in each system and that a great deal of the difference between these apparently opposed methods of treatment lies in the claims of their exponents. It will be shown presently that, in their final analysis, the osteopathic spinal lesion, the chiropractic subluxation and the naprapathic ligatight represent one and the same thing.

Natural Therapeutics is broad enough to embrace all methods of treatment, no matter what their source, provided they harmonize with the fundamental laws of cure.

Gradually, therefore, after having gathered the **constructive** elements from **all** the various methods of manipulation, after considerable spinal dissection and, above all, after close observation of the results obtained in hundreds of obstinate acute and chronic cases, we of the School of Natural Therapeutics have evolved our own system of spinal manipulation and have named it **neurotherapy.**

The Relation of Neurotherapy to Other Manipulative Systems

Osteopathy, chiropractic, naprapathy, neurotherapy and spondylotherapy, as we have learned, are various systems of maipulative treatment which have been devised mainly to correct spinal and other bony lesions, shrinkage and contracture of muscles, ligaments and other connective tissues.

Important as these methods are in the treatment of acute and chronic diseases, by themselves they are not all-sufficient because they deal only with the mechanical causes of disease, not with the chemical, thermal or with the mental and psychical. The most efficient spinal treatment cannot make good for the **bad effects of an unbalanced diet** which contains an excessive amount of poison-producing materials and is deficient in the all-important mineral elements or organic salts. Just as surely as mental therapeutics and a natural diet cannot correct bony lesions produced by external violence, just so surely is it impossible to cure dementia praecox, monomania or obsession, or to supply iron, lime, sodium, etc., to the system by correcting spinal lesions.

The trouble with the manipulative schools and their graduates is that they adhere too closely to the mechanical theory and treatment of disease; that they reject practically all natural methods of treatment aside from manipulative and that so far as the osteopathic school is concerned its practitioners show a strong tendency to fall back upon the "Old School" methods of drugging and of surgical treatment. This is due to the fact that in many types of diseases manipulative treatment by itself has proved insufficient to produce satisfactory results.

In order to do justice to our patients and not neglect our responsibilities toward them **we must use in the treatment of disease all that is good in all the natural methods of healing.** In serious chronic cases any single one of these methods, whether it be pure food diet, hydrotherapy, massage, spinal treatment, mental therapeutics or homeopathy, is not by itself sufficient to achieve satisfactory results or to produce them fast enough.

To use an illustration: Suppose a wagon full of freight requires the combined strength of six horses to move it and suppose that number of horses is available, would it not be foolish to try to move the load with one, two, three, four or even five horses? Would not common sense suggest the saving of time and effort by putting all six horses to work at once?

In Natural Therapeutics every one of the various methods of treatment is supplemented and assisted by all the others.

The manipulative schools of healing maintain that practically all disease is caused by mechanical abnormalities of the spinal column or of muscles, ligaments and other connective tissues, due to abnormal strain or injury. The philosophy of Natural Therapeutics, on the other hand, points out that a large percentage of such spinal and other mechanical lesions are secondary manifestations of disease, not primary causes; that acute or subacute inflammatory conditions in the interior of the body may cause nervous irritation and thereby contraction of muscles and ligaments and, as a result of these, subluxations of vertebrae or of other bony structures.

The naprapathic theory of disease postulates that it is the shrinkage and contraction of the connective tissues, which serve as a support and protection for the nerve matter contained in the nerve trunks and filaments, that cause interference with the normal nerve supply of cells and tissues and thereby abnormal function and disease.

The philosophy of Natural Therapeutics points to the fact that this shrinkage and contraction of the connective tissues surrounding and permeating the nerve trunks and filaments is caused by certain acids and other pathogenic materials which are produced by faulty diet and defective elimination and that the same causes produce accumulation of waste and morbid matter in the tissues of the body which, all through the system, interfere just as effectually with nutrition, drainage and innervation of the cells and tissue as do spinal lesions and ligatights.

While the other systems of manipulative treatment confine themselves almost entirely to the correction of bony and other connective tissue lesions, to "pressing the button," as it is called, neurotherapy, besides this, aims at other very important results.

In disease the tissues are either in an abnormally tense and contracted or in a weak, relaxed condition. The functional activities are either hyperactive as in acute inflammation, or sluggish and inactive as in chronic atonic and atrophic conditions. These extremes can be powerfully influenced and equalized by manipulative inhibition, relaxation or stimulation.

During an acute attack of gastritis, for instance, the neurotherapist would exert strong inhibition on the nerves which supply the stomach. This is accomplished by deep and persistent pressure on the nerves where they emerge from the spinal openings (foramina). This diminishes the rush of blood and nerve currents to the inflamed organ and thereby eases but does not suppress the inflammatory process and the attending congestion and pain.

In case of extreme tension in any part of the system, relaxation of the shrunken tissues can be brought about by gentle but persistent stretching of the nerves and adjacent muscles and ligaments, in a manner similar to that of the naprapathic directos.

When the vital organs and their functions are weak and inactive or when nerves, muscles, ligaments and other connective tissues are in a relaxed, atonic or atrophic condition, certain stimulating movements applied to the nerves where they emerge from the spinal column will energize the vital functions all through the system.

Many patients imagine that such manipulative treatment is superficial. To them it is just "rubbing" and seems all alike. They do not realize that manipulative stimulation applied to the nerves near the surface of the body travels all along their branches and filaments like electricity along a complicated system of copper wires and thus reaches the innermost cells and organs of the body, making them more alive and active. This internal stimulation of vital activities is attained also by good massage through energizing the nerve endings all over the surface of the body.

The Fundamental Difference Between Neuratherapy and Other Manipulative Systems

The following paragraphs will explain the fundamental difference between neurotherapy and the older systems of manipulative treatment. The older systems, the same as the allopathic school of medicine, look upon acute diseases as destructive processes dangerous to health and life; therefore they endeavor to check or suppress them as quickly as possible by their various methods.

Neurotherapy so far is the only system of manipulative treatment that bases its work on the fundamental laws of Natural Therapeutics. According to these laws every acute disease is the result of a purifying, healing effort of Nature. Therefore neurotherapy would not suppress acute processes by manipulative treatment any more than by drugs, ice, antitoxins, surgery or any other suppressive method.

To illustrate: Supposing that spontaneously or as a result of natural living and treatment a patient suffering from chronic constipation, indigestion, etc., develops a vigorous purging, which we of the Nature Cure school would consider a splendid healing crisis. Under allopathic as well as under the treatment of other manipulative schools such an acute reaction would be immediately suppressed. This can be accomplished very easily by a few manipulative moves, but it would mean the suppression of a purifying healing crisis and this would result in throwing the patient back into his old chronic condition. The underlying causes of disease must be removed before we can cure chronic disease and bring about a normal condition of the organism.

Suppose manipulative treatment should succeed in stopping a fever instantaneously. This would suppress Nature's purifying, regenerating efforts, the patient would continue to "load up" more morbid materials (especially since these schools do not teach the importance of natural living) and it would only be a matter of time until the morbid accumulations in the body would excite new acute reactions, necessitating more adjustments. This may be all right for the practitioner; but what about the patient? In the long run it can only have one result, and that is chronic disease.

Chapter XXXIII

Legitimate Scope and Natural Limitations
of Mental and Metaphysical Healing

During the last generation people have perceived more or less clearly the fallacies of "Old School" medicine and surgery. They have grown more and more suspicious of orthodox theories and practices. From allopathic "overdoing" the pendulum has swung to the other extreme of metaphysical nihilism, to the "underdoing" of mental and metaphysical systems of treating human ailments.

Some of these systems and cults of metaphysical healing have met with success and wide popularity and this is looked upon by their followers as a proof that all the claims and teachings of these cults and isms are based upon absolute truth.

However, a thorough understanding of the fundamental Laws of Cure, as I have explained them in this volume, will reveal in how far their teachings and their practices are based upon truth and in how far they are inspired by erroneous assumptions.

Let us then apply the yardstick and the weights and measures of Nature Cure philosophy in testing the true value of the claims of metaphysical healers.

For ages people have been educated in the belief that almost every acute disease will end fatally unless the patient is drugged or operated on. When they find to their surprise that the metaphysical formulas or prayers of a mental healer or Christian Scientist will "cure" baby's measles or father's smallpox just as well as, and possibly better than, Dr. Dopem's pills and potions, they are firmly convinced that a miracle has been performed in their behalf and straightway they become blind believers in and fanatical followers of their new idols.

They simply exchange one superstition for another: the belief in the efficacy of drugs and surgical operations for the belief in the wonder-working power of a metaphysical formula, a self-appointed savior or a reason-stultifying and will-benumbing cult. They have not been taught that **every acute disease is the result of a healing effort of Nature** and therefore fail to see that it is **vital force,** the physician within, that, if conditions are favorable, cures measles and smallpox as easily as it repairs the broken blade of grass or heals the wounded deer of the forest.

"That is exactly what we say," exclaim healer and scientist. "Have unlimited faith in the God within and all will be well."

True, faith is good, but faith and works are better. Though we cannot heal and give life, we can in many ways assist the healer within. We can teach and explain Nature's Laws, we can remove obstructions and we can make the conditions within and around the patient more favorable for the action of Nature's healing forces.

When the Great Master said: "Go forth and sin no more, lest worse things than these befall you," he acknowledged sin, or the transgression of natural laws, to be the primary cause of disease, and made health dependent upon compliance with the Law. The necessity of complying with the Law, in all respects and on all the planes of being, is still more strongly emphasized in the following:

> "For whosoever shall keep the whole law and yet offend in one point, he is guilty of all."

The skeptic and the superficial reader may reply: "This saying is utterly unreasonable. Stealing a penny is not committing a murder; overeating does not break the law of chastity; how, then, is it possible to break all laws by breaking any single one of them?" There is, however, a deeper meaning to this seeming paradox which makes it scientifically true.

Self-Control, the Whole Law

Obedience to all laws on all planes of being depends primarily on self-control. Self-control is, therefore, in a sense, the whole law, for man cannot break any one law unless he breaks first this fundamental Law of all Laws. This implies that the demoralizing effect of sinning or lawbreaking, on any one of the planes of being, does not depend so much upon the enormity of the deed as upon the loss of self-control. Continued weakening of self-control in trivial things may therefore, in the end, prove more destructive than a murder committed in the heat of passion. If there is not self-control enough to resist a cup of coffee or a cigar, whence shall come the will-power to resist greater temptations?

Truly, lack of self-control in small things is the "dry rot" of the soul. Is it not, then, somewhat unreasonable to expect God or Nature to strain and twist the immutable laws of Nature at the request of every healer in order to save us from the natural consequences of overeating, red meat eating, whisky drinking, smoking, tobacco chewing, drugging and a thousand and one other transgressions of natural laws?

In spite of the finest-spun metaphysical sophistries, we continue to burn our fingers in the fire until we know enough to leave it alone. Herein lies the corrective purpose of that which we call evil—suffering and disease. The rational thing to do is not to deny the existence of Mother Nature's punishing rod, but to escape her salubrious spankings by conforming to her Laws.

What about the "Cures"?

As in medicine, so also in metaphysical healing, men judge by superficial results, not by the real underlying causes. The usual answer to any criticism of Christian Science or kindred methods of cure is: "That may be all right; but see the results! Nobody can deny their wonderful cures," etc.

Let us see whether there really is anything wonderful or supernatural about these cures or whether they can be explained on simple, natural grounds.

In another chapter we explain the difference between functional and organic disease and show how in diseases of the functional type the life force or healing force, which always endeavors to establish normal conditions and the perfect type, may work unaided up to the reconstructive healing crises and through these eliminate the morbid encumbrances from the system and reestablish normal structure and function.

It is in cases like these that metaphysicians attain their best results simply because **Nature helps herself.**

On the other hand, in cases of the true **organic** type, where the vitality is low and the destruction of vital parts and organs has progressed to a considerable extent, the system is no longer able to arouse itself to self-help.

In such cases, faith alone is not sufficient to obtain results. It must be backed and assisted by all the natural methods of treatment at our command.

Healers Work with Laws that They Do Not Understand

In our critical analysis of "Old School" methods we found that by far the greater part of all chronic ailments is due to drugging and to surgery. People commence doctoring for little troubles, which are aggravated by every dose of medicine and every surgical operation until they end in big troubles.

Is it marvelous that such patients improve and that many are cured when they are weaned from drugs and the knife?

Metaphysical healers unwittingly do their best and most beneficial work because they induce their followers not to suppress acute diseases and healing crises by drugs and surgical operations, thus allowing them to run their natural course in harmony with the fundamental law of Nature Cure, which states that every acute disease is the result of a cleansing and healing effort of Nature. People will refrain from the suppressive drug treatment under the influence of metaphysical teachings, which appeal to the miracle-loving element in their nature, when they cannot be convinced by common sense Nature Cure reasoning.

Thus metaphysicians assist Nature indirectly by noninterference and directly by soothing fear and worry, by instilling faith, hope and confidence. Frequently they also aid Nature by prohibiting the use of tobacco, alcohol and pork, and by regulating otherwise the life and habits of their followers.

Let us consider the problem from another point of view. Let us assume, for argument's sake, that the average person passes in the course of a lifetime through a dozen different diseases. He recovers from eleven of these, no matter what the treatment. It is only the twelfth to which he succumbs. Yet, whosoever happened to treat the first eleven diseases claims to have **cured** them and, perhaps, to have saved the patient's life when, as a matter of fact, he recovered very often in spite of the treatment and not because of it.

These explanations account for the seemingly miraculous results of metaphysical healing. If healers and Christian Scientists were to explain their cures by the laws and principles of Nature Cure philosophy, mystery and miracle would be taken out of their business.

"Faith Without Works" Is Dangerous

To believe that God or Nature will overcome the natural effects of our ignorance, laziness and viciousness by wonders, signs and metaphysics, or to deny the existence of sickness, sin and suffering, must lead inevitably to intellectual and moral stagnation and degeneration. I am a thorough and consistent optimist and New Thought enthusiast, but I do not overlook the fact that in this, as in everything else, there lurks always the danger of overdoing and of exaggerating virtue into fault.

The greatest danger of this revulsion from old-time pessimism to modern optimism lies in the fact that the Higher Thought enthusiast may cut from under his feet the solid ground of reality; that he may become a dreamer instead of a thinker and doer; and that he may mistake selfish, emotional sentimentalism for practical charity and altruism.

This unhealthy "all-is-good, there-is-no-evil" emotionalism leads only too often to weakening of personal effort, a deadening of the sense of individual responsibility and thereby to mental and moral atrophy; for any of our voluntary functions, capacities and powers which we fail to exercise will in time become benumbed and paralyzed. Unprejudiced observers who come in close contact with metaphysicians cannot help perceiving the pernicious effect of their subtle sophistries on reason and character.

A chronic invalid who had been under the treatment of a faith healer for several years exclaimed, when we gave her our various instructions for dieting, bathing, breathing exercises, etc.: "How glad I am that you give me something to do! **I fear I have been imposing too long on the goodness of the Lord, expecting Him to do my work for me.**" Often afterwards, while recovering from lifelong ailments, she expressed her happiness and contentment in that she herself was doing something which in her opinion was rational and helpful because it assisted Nature's healing efforts.

We believe firmly and fully in the influence of mind over matter, in the fact that vibrations of the physical plane by continuity create corresponding vibrations on the mental and psychical planes and vice versa. We know that, in accordance with this law, anything which affects the mind or the moral life of a person affects also his physical condition; but instead of hypnotizing the minds of our patients by law-defying, reason- and will-benumbing dogmas and formulas, we strengthen and harmonize their mental vibrations by appealing to reason, by teaching and explaining natural laws instead of obscuring and denying them.

The more intelligent the patient, the more amenable he will be to such normal suggestions based on scientific truth and on the dictates of reason and common sense.

While nonresistance to Nature's healing efforts is better than suppression by drugs or the knife, there is something more helpful and rational than the negative attitude toward disease on the physical plane assumed by metaphysical healing cults. **That "something" is intelligent cooperation with Nature's cleansing and healing efforts.**

Where the Old School fails by sins of commission, the Faith Schools fail by sins of omission. Many patients are sacrificed daily through fanatical inactivity, when their lives might be saved by a wet pack or a cold sponge bath, by an internal bath, rational diet, judicious fasting, scientific manipulation or some other simple yet powerful remedy of natural healing. To permit a patient to perish in a burning fever, depending solely upon the efficacy of prayers, formulas and mental attitude, when wet packs and cold sponging would in a few minutes reduce the temperature below the danger point, is manslaughter, even though it be done in the name of religion.

Incidents like the following are common in our practice: A little girl in the neighborhood of our institution was taken with diphtheria. The mother, an ardent Christian Scientist, called in several healers of her cult, but the child grew worse from day to day, until the false membranes in the throat began to choke her to death.

A boarder in the house, who was a follower of Nature Cure, finally induced the mother to call upon us for advice by threatening to notify the City Health Department. Within an hour after the application of the whole-body packs and the cold ablutions, the blood was sufficiently drawn away from the local congestion in the throat into the surface of the body, so that the child breathed easily and freely, and from then on made a splendid recovery.

Another instance: A man had been suffering from sciatic rheumatism for fifteen years. He had swallowed poisonous drugs to no avail. For several years he had been under Mental Science treatment, but the suffering had grown more intense.

When he applied to us for help, we found that the right hip bone (the innominate) had slipped upward and backward. A few manipulative treatments replaced the bone where it belonged, and the sciatic rheumatism was cured.

In this case, the combined concentration and prayers of all the metaphysical healers on earth would not have succeeded in replacing the dislocated hip bone, which required the full strength of a trained manipulator.

Metaphysicians could not have accomplished this feat any more than they could have moved, by their mental efforts, a hundred-pound weight from one place to another. Mechanical lesions of that kind (and there are many of them) require mechanical treatment.

Another factor which makes converts to metaphysical healing cults by the hundreds and thousands is the get-rich-quick instinct in human nature, the desire to get something for nothing, or with as little effort as possible. Herein lies the seductive pull of old-time drugging and of modern metaphysics. "It does not matter how you live; when you get into trouble, a bottle of medicine or a metaphysical formula will make it all right." That sounds very easy and promising, but the trouble is—it does not always work.

Our forefathers were too pessimistic; higher thought enthusiasts are often too optimistic. While the former poisoned their lives and paralyzed their God-given faculties and powers by dismal dread of hell's fire and damnation, our modern healers and Scientists have drifted to the other extreme. They tell us there is no sin, no pain, no suffering. If that be true, there is also no action and reaction, no Law of Compensation, no personal responsibility, no need of self-control, self-help or personal effort.

The ideal of the faith healer is the ideal of the animal. The animal trusts implicitly, it has absolute faith; guided by instinct, God, or Nature, it follows the promptings of its appetites and passions without worrying about right or wrong. It acts today as it did ten thousand years ago.

In man, **reason** has taken the place of instinct; we must think and manage for ourselves. We are free and responsible moral agents. If we deny this, we deny the very foundations of equity, justice and right. It behooves us to use the talents which God has given us, to study the laws of our being and to comply with them to the best of our ability, so that enlightened reason may take the place of animal instinct and guide us to physical, mental and moral perfection.

Chapter XXXIV

The Difference Between Functional and Organic Disease

Much confusion concerning the curability of chronic diseases by the various methods of treatment arises because people do not understand the difference between **functional** and **organic** chronic disease.

For instance, there is a close resemblance between pseudo- and true locomotor ataxy. Often it is difficult to distinguish functional lung trouble from the organic type of the disease. In our practice, several cases of mental derangement which had been diagnosed as true paresis proved to be of the functional type and under natural treatment recovered rapidly.

Functional diseases may present a very serious appearance and may be labeled with awe-inspiring Greek or Latin names, and yet yield readily to natural methods of living and treatment.

In diseases of an **organic** nature, however, right living and self-treatment are usually not sufficient to obtain satisfactory results. In such cases all forms of active and passive treatment must be applied, and even then it is frequently difficult and sometimes impossible to produce a cure.

Chronic diseases of a functional nature develop when an otherwise healthy organism becomes saturated and clogged with food and drug poisons to such an extent that these encumbrances interfere with the free circuation of the blood and nerve currents, and with the normal functions of the cells, organs and tissues of the body.

Such cases resemble a watch which is losing time because its works are filled with dust. All that such a waste-encumbered watch or body needs, in order to restore normal functions, is a good cleaning. Pure food diet, fasting, systematic exercise, deep breathing, cold bathing and the right mental attitude are usually sufficient to perform this physical housecleaning and to restore perfect health.

Functional disorders yield readily to the various forms of metaphysical treatment. Remove such patients from the weakening and destructive effects of poisonous drugs and of surgical operations, supplant fear and worry by courage and faith, and the results often seem miraculous to those who do not understand the power of the purifying and stimulating influence of clean living and of the right mental attitude.

In diseases of the **organic** type, however, good results are not so easily achieved. A body affected by organic disease resembles a watch whose mechanism has been injured and partly destroyed by rust and corrosive acids. If such be the case, cleaning and oiling alone will not be sufficient to put the timepiece in good working order. The watchmaker has to replace the damaged parts.

This is easy enough in the case of the watch, but it is not so easily accomplished in the human body. Besides, in many instances the corroding acids are the very medicines which were given to cure the disease and the injury and destruction of vital parts and organs is only too often the direct or indirect result of surgical operations.

The watchmaker may remove those parts of the watch which are suffering from organic trouble, and replace them by new ones. This the surgeon cannot do. He can extirpate, but he cannot replace. Operative treatment leaves the organism forever after in a mutilated and therefore unbalanced condition, and often prevents and frustrates Nature's cleansing and healing crises.

The Limitations of Metaphysical Healing

In the writings of metaphysical healers we often meet the assertion that they can cure organic diseases as easily and quickly as functional ailments. If they understood better the difference between functional and organic disorders as explained in the foregoing pages, they would not make such deceptive and extravagant claims. They would then realize the natural limitations of metaphysical healing.

°I do not underestimate the great value of mental, metaphysical and spiritual healing methods. Of these I shall speak more fully in subsequent chapters. But I do claim that we can and should aid Nature's healing efforts not only by the right mental attitude and the prayer of faith, but also by natural living and many different methods of physical treatment.

Mental attitude alone will not clean the watch. To concentrate on the work of housecleaning without using broom, soap and water is not sufficient. Reason and common sense teach us that the removal of physical, material encumbrances can be, to say the least, accelerated by the use of physical or physiological agents. Anyone who has observed or himself experienced the efficacy of natural diet, cold-water treatment, massage and osteopathy in dealing with the morbid accumulations in the system will never again underestimate the practical value of these "brooms."

In our study of the nature and purpose of acute diseases we have found that Nature tries to purify the system from its morbid encumbrances through inflammatory, febrile processes (acute diseases) and that these cleansing efforts of Nature are generally prevented, checked and suppressed by allopathic methods of medical and surgical treatment, and thus changed into chronic disease conditions.

The metaphysical healers do away with these suppressive methods of treatment and allow Nature's acute cleansing and healing efforts to run their natural course. Thus they profit by the fundamental laws of cure without understanding them. **The acute disease, whose very existence they deny, is in reality the cure.**

Furthermore, rational mental and metaphysical treatment supports Nature's efforts **actively** by supplanting the weakening and paralyzing fear vibrations with relaxing and invigorating vibrations of hope, confidence and faith in the supremacy of Nature's healing forces. Under these favorable conditions, the organism will arouse itself to the purifying and constructive healing crises (the chemicalizations of Christian Science) and through these eliminate the morbid encumbrances and restore normal structure and functions.

°While functional disorders, in nearly every case, yield readily enough to the natural methods of living and of treatment and to the right mental attitude, it is different with organic diseases.

When waste matter, ptomaines or poisonous alkaloids and acids produced in the body as a result of wrong diet and other violations of Nature's laws have brought about destruction and corrosion in vital parts and organs—when dislocations and subluxations of bony structures, or new growths and accumulations in the forms of tumors, stones or gravel obstruct the blood vessels and nerve currents, shut off the supply of the vital fluids and thus cause malnutrition and gradual decay of the tissues—when, in addition to this, the organism has been poisoned or mutilated by drugs and surgical operations, then its purification and repair becomes a tedious and difficult task.

Not only must the mechanism of the body be cleansed and freed from obstructive and destructive materials, but the injured parts must be repaired, morbid growths and abnormal formations dissolved and eliminated and lesions in the bony structures corrected by manipulative treatment.

In organic diseases, the vitality is usually so low and destruction so great that the organism cannot arouse itself to self-help. Even the cessation of suppressive treatment and the stimulating influence of mental and metaphysical therapeutics are not sufficient to bring about the reconstructive healing crises. **This can only be accomplished by the combined influences of all the natural methods of living and of treatment.**

It is in cases like these that metaphysical healing and hygienic living find their limitations. Such organic defects require systematic treatment by all the methods, active and passive, which the best Nature Cure sanitariums can furnish. It may be slow and laborious work to obtain satisfactory results, and if the vitality is too low or the destruction of vital parts and organs has too far advanced, even the best and most complete combination of natural methods of treatment may fail to produce a cure.

However, this can be determined only by a fair trial of the natural methods. The forces of Nature are ever ready to react to persistent, systematic effort in the right direction and when there is enough vitality to keep alive there is likely to be enough to purify and reconstruct the organism and in time to bring about improvement and cure.

This, then, explains why, in the organic types of diseases, metaphysical methods of treatment alone are insufficient. At least one-half of the patients that come to the Nature Cure physician have faithfully tried these methods without avail, but the failures are easily excused by lack of faith, wrong mental attitude or something wrong with the patient or his surroundings.

In our experience with patients who had formerly tried metaphysical methods of healing faithfully, but without results, we sometimes come face to face with a curious and amusing phase of human nature. As our patients improve under the natural regimen and treatment, they gradually return to their first love and ascribe the good effects of natural treatment to a better understanding of "the Science." As health and strength return, they say: "Formerly I did not know just how to apply the Science, but now I know, and that is why I am growing better."

I suppose this form of self-deception which we have frequently observed is due to the fact that people feel flattered by the idea that Providence has taken a special interest in their case and cured them by miraculous intervention. It is so much more interesting to be cured by some occult principle than by diet and cold water.

Undoubtedly it is this miracle-loving element in human nature that makes metaphysical healing so much more popular than plain, commonsense Nature Cure.

Not long ago Professor Münsterberg investigated the claims of Christian Scientists that they were constantly curing diseases of the organic type. He reported his findings in a series of articles in McClure's Magazine (1908), stating that he inquired personally into one hundred cases said to have been cured by Christian Science and found that ninety-two of them had been of the functional type, while eight were claimed to have been organic, but that in no instance could this be proved beyond doubt.

Chapter XXXV

The Two-fold Attitude of Mind and Soul

The following is an extract from a letter sent to me by a reader of my articles in *The Nature Cure Magazine*.

"Sometimes you say we must rely on our own personal efforts and at other times you teach dependence upon a higher power. This, to me, is contradictory and confusing. I cannot understand how, consistently, we can do both at the same time. Which is right? Is it best to rely upon our own power and our personal efforts or upon the 'Higher Power'?"

Similar inquiries have come from other friends. I shall now endeavor to answer these and other questions.

There is nothing contradictory or incompatible in the teachings of the Nature Cure philosophy concerning the physical and metaphysical methods of treating human ailments. Both the independent and the dependent attitudes of mind and soul are good and true and may be entertained at the same time. It is necessary for us to rely on our own personal efforts in carrying out the dictates of reason and of common sense. But this need not prevent us from praying for and confidently expecting a larger inflow of vital power and intuitional discernment from the Source of all intelligence and power in the innermost parts of our being.

This two-fold attitude of mind and soul is justified not only by reason and intuition, but also by the anatomical structure of the human organism and its physiological and psychological faculties, capacities and powers.

The activities of the human organism are governed by two different systems of nerves, the sympathetic and the motor. The sympathetic nervous system is the conveyor of vital force to the organs and cells of the body. Just what this vital force is and where it ultimately comes from, we do not know. It is a manifestation of that which we call God, Nature, Life, the Higher Power or the Divine Within.

Heart action, the circulation of the blood, respiration, digestion, assimilation of food, elimination and all other involuntary activities and functions of the human organism are controlled by means of the sympathetic nervous system. The nature of the controlling force itself is not known to us. We do know that it is supremely powerful, intelligent and benevolent.

The more we study the anatomy, physiology and psychology of the human organism, the more we wonder at its marvelous complexity and ingenuity of structure and function. Every moment there are enacted in our bodies innumerable mechanical, chemical and psychological miracles. Who, or what, performs these miracles? We do not know. Yet every moment of our lives depends upon the infinite care and wisdom of this unknown intelligence and power.

Why, then, should we not trust the One so faithful? Why should we not ask aid from One so powerful? Why not seek enlightenment from One who is so wise and so benevolent?

However, not all of the human entity is dependent upon a controlling power, nor are all its functions involuntary. Within the house prepared by the Divine Intelligence, there dwells a sovereign in his own right and by his own might. He is endowed with freedom of desire, of choice and of action. He creates in his brain the nerve centers which control the voluntary activities of the body and from these brain centers he sends his commands through the fibers of the motor nerves to the voluntary muscles and makes them do his bidding; some he commands to walk, others to laugh, to eat, to speak, etc.

This independent principle in man we call the ego, the individual intelligence. It imagines, desires, reasons, plans and works out, by the power of free will and independent choice, its own salvation or destruction, physically, mentally, morally and spiritually. By means of the motor nervous system, this thinker and doer directs and controls from the headquarters in the brain all the voluntary functions, capacities and powers of the human organism.

This part of the human entity can evolve and progress only through its own conscious and voluntary personal efforts.

In this, Man differs from the animal creation. The animal is able to take care of itself shortly after birth. It inherits, already fully developed, those brain centers for the control of the bodily functions which the newborn human must develop slowly and laboriously through patient and persistent effort in the course of many years.

Of voluntary capacities and powers the newborn infant possesses little more than the simplest unicellular animalcule, that is, about all it can do is to scent and swallow food. Its cerebral hemispheres are as yet blank slates, to be inscribed gradually by its conscious and voluntary exertions. Before it can think, reason, speak, walk or do anything else, it must first develop in its brain special centers for each and every one of these voluntary faculties and functions.

Through these persistent personal efforts, reason, will and self-control are gradually evolved and developed; while the animal, being hereditarily endowed with the faculties and functions necessary for the maintenance of life, has no occasion for the development of the **higher** faculties and powers and therefore remains an irresponsible automaton, which cannot be held accountable for its actions.

To recapitulate: Freedom of choice and of action distinguish the human from the animal. In the animal kingdom, reasoning power and freedom of action move in the narrow limits of heredity and instinct, while Man, through his own personal efforts, is capable of unlimited development physically, mentally, morally and spiritually, both here and hereafter. We say physically advisedly, for in the spiritual realms, in the life after death, the physical (spiritual-material) body also is capable of deterioration or of ever greater refinement and beautification.

Through the right use of his voluntary faculties, capacities and powers, Man is enabled to become the master of himself and of his destiny.

Thus we find that the human organism consists of two distinct parts or departments, the one acting independently of the ego and deriving its motive force from an unknown source and the other under the conscious and voluntary control of the ego.

This two-fold nature of the human entity justifies the two-fold attitude of mind and soul, on the one hand the prayerful and faithful dependence upon that mysterious power which flows into us and controls us through the sympathetic nervous system and on the other hand the conscious and voluntary dominion over the various faculties, capacities and powers with which Nature has endowed us.

It is our privilege and our duty to maintain both attitudes, the dependent as well as the independent. The desire and the will to plan, to choose and to perform are ours, but for the power to execute we are dependent upon a Higher Source.

Chapter XXXVI

The Symphony of Life

Human life appears to me as a great orchestra in which we are the players. The great composition to be performed is the "Symphony of Life," its infinitude of dissonances and melodies blending into one colossal tone picture of harmony and grandeur. We players must study the laws of music and the score of the Great Symphony and we must practice diligently and persistently, until we can play our part unerringly in harmony with the concepts of the Great Composer. At the same time we must learn to keep our instrument, the body, in the best possible condition; for the greatest artist, endowed with a profound knowledge of the laws of music and possessed of the most perfect technique, cannot produce musical and harmonious sounds from an instrument with strings relaxed or overtense, or with its body filled with rubbish.

The artist must learn that the instrument, its material, its construction and its care are just as subject to law as the harmonics of the score.

In the final analysis, everything is vibration acting in and on the universal ethers, which are held to be the primordial substance. Possibly the ethers themselves are modes of vibration.

That which is constructive is harmonious vibration. That which is destructive is inharmonious or discordant vibration.

Against this it may be urged that devolution has its harmonics as well as evolution, that every symphony is made up of dissonances as well as of harmonies. To this I answer: "Unadulterated harmony may, solely for lack of change, become monotonous; but discords alone never create melody, harmony, health or happiness."

As the artist seeks vibratory harmony between his instrument and the harmonics of the universe of sound, so the health-seeker must endeavor to establish vibratory unison between the material elements of his body and Nature's harmonics of health in the physical universe.

The atoms and molecules in the wood and strings of the violin, as well as the sounds produced from them, are modes of motion or vibration. In order to bring forth musical and harmonious notes, the vibratory conditions of the physical elements of the violin must be in harmonious vibratory relationship with Nature's harmonics in the universe of sound.

The elements and forces composing the human body are also vibratory in their nature, the same as the material elements of the violin. They also must be kept in a certain well-balanced chemical combination, mechanical adjustment and physical refinement before they can vibrate in unison with Nature's harmonics in the physical universe and thus produce the harmonies of health and strength and beauty.

If our instrument is out of tune, or if we ignorantly or willfully insist on playing in our own way, regardless of the score, we create discords not only for ourselves, but also for our fellow artists in the great orchestra of life.

Sin, disease, suffering and evil are nothing but discords, produced by the ignorance, indifference or malice of the players.Therefore we cannot attribute the discords of life to the Great Composer. They are of our own making and will last as long as we refuse to learn our parts and to play them in tune with the Great Score. For in this way only can we ever hope to master the art and science of right living and to enjoy the harmonies of peace, self-content and happiness.

Chapter XXXVII

The Three-fold Constitution of Man

he following diagram and accompanying explanations will serve to illustrate "Three Planes of Being," the corresponding "Three-fold Constitution of man," and their analogy to the artist and his instrument.

The Three-fold Constitution of Man

Planes of Being	Three-fold Constitution of Man	Analogy
Psychical or Moral	Soul	Music, Laws of Harmony
Mental	Mind	Player
Material	Bodies (Physical and Spiritual)	Violin

Man lives and functions on three distinct planes of being: the physical-material and spiritual-material, the mental and the soul (psychical or moral) planes.

He may be diseased upon any one or more of these planes. The true physician must look for causes of disease and for methods of treatment upon all three planes of being.

The purely materialistic physician concentrates all his study and effort upon the physical-material plane of being. To him, mental, spiritual, psychical, and moral phenomena are merely chemical and physiological actions and reactions of brain and nerve substance. He has nothing but contempt and derision for the man who believes in or knows of a spiritual body or a soul.

He is like an artist who says: "My violin is all there is to music. The musician's art consists in keeping his instrument in good condition. Technique and the laws of harmony are a matter of imagination and of superstitious belief."

On the other hand, mental healers, Christian Scientists and faith healers concentrate all their efforts upon either the mental or the soul plane, frequently making no distinction between the two. In the treatment of disease, they ignore the conditions and needs of the physical body, and some of them even deny its existence.

These metaphysicians are like the artist who devotes all his time and energy to the study and practice of technique, counterpoint and harmony, neglecting his instrument and taking no heed whether its mechanism is out of order or its interior filled with rubbish. His knowledge of the laws of harmonics and his execution may be ever so perfect; but with his instrument out of tune and out of order he will produce discords instead of harmony.

The true artist realizes that **MIND**, the **player**, must study **SOUL**, the **harmonics;** and that the mind must also have its **instrument**, the **BODY**, in perfect condition in order to interpret perfectly and artistically the harmonies of the symphony of life. Likewise, the Nature Cure physician will look for causes of disease and for means of cure upon the material, mental and psychical planes of being.

Thus will higher civilization and greater knowledge lead back to the natural simplicity of primitive races, where physician and priest are one.

After all, physical health is the best possible basis for the attainment of mental, moral and spiritual health. All building begins with the foundation. We do not first suspend the steeple in the air and then build the church under it. So also, the building of the temple of human character should begin by laying the foundation in physical health.

We have known people who had attained high intellectual, moral and spiritual development and then suffered utter shipwreck physically, mentally and in every other way, because ignorantly they had violated the laws of their physical nature.

There are others who believe that the possession of occult knowledge and the achievement of mastership confer absolute control over Nature's forces and phenomena on the physical plane. These people believe that a man is not a master if he does not miraculously heal all manner of disease and raise the dead.

If such things were possible, they would overthrow the Laws of Cause and Effect and of Compensation. They would abolish the basic principles of morality and constructive spirituality. If it is possible in one case to heal disease and to overcome death through the fiat of the will of a master, then it must be possible in all cases. If so, then we can ignore the existence of Nature's laws, indulge our appetites and passions to the fullest extent, and when the natural results of our transgressions overtake us, we can go to a healer or master and have our diseases instantly and painlessly removed, like a bad tooth.

I say this with all due reverence for, and faith in, the efficacy of true prayer and with full knowledge of the healing power of therapeutic faith, but I do not believe that God, or Nature, or a master or metaphysical formulas can or will make good in a miraculous way for the inevitable results of our transgressions of the natural laws that govern our being.

If such miraculous healing were possible and of common occurrence, what occasion would there be for the exercise of reason, will and self-control? What would become of the scientific basis of morality and constructive spirituality?

All this leads us to the following conclusions:

"If there is in operation a constructive principle of Nature on the ethical, moral and spiritual planes of being, with which we must align ourselves and to which we must conform our conscious and voluntary activities in order to achieve self-completion, self-content, individual completion and happiness, then this constructive principle must be in operation also in our physical bodies and in their corelated physical, mental and emotional activities. If the constructive principle is active in the physical as well as in the moral and spiritual realms, then the established harmonic relationship of the physical to the constructive law of its being must constitute the morality of the physical; and from this it follows that the achievement of health on the physical plane is as much under our conscious and voluntary control as the working out of our individual salvation on the higher planes of life."

To recapitulate:

First, our well-being on all planes and in all relationships of life depends upon the existence, recognition and practical application of the great fundamental laws and principles just explained.

Second: Physical health, as well as moral health, is of our own making. We are personally responsible not only for our own physical and mental health, but we are also morally responsible for the hereditary tendencies of our offspring toward health or disease.

Third: The attainment of physical health through compliance with Nature's laws is just as much a part of the Great Work as our ethical, moral and psychical development.

The Unity and Continuity of the Law

That which we call God, Nature, the Creator or the Universal Intelligence is the great central cause of all things and the vibratory activities produced by or proceeding from this central or primary cause continue through all spheres of life, in like manner as the light waves of the sun, moon and fixed stars penetrate through the intervening spheres of life to our plane of earth. Therefore all powers, forces, laws and principles which manifest on our plane proceed and continue from the innermost Divine to the most external plane in physical nature. This explains the continuity, stability and correspondence on all planes of being of that which we call Natural Law. In other words, **"Natural Law is the established harmonic relationship of effects and phenomena to their causes and of all particular causes to the one great primary cause of all things."**

Chapter XXXVIII

Mental Therapeutics

The new psychology and the science of mental and spiritual healing teach us that the lower principles in Man stand or should stand under the dominion of the higher. The physical body, with its material elements, is dominated and guided by the mind. The mind is inspired through the inner consciousness, which is an attribute of the soul. The soul of man is in communion with the Oversoul, which is the Source of all life and all intelligence animating the universe.

Wherever this natural order is reversed, there is discord or disease. Too many people think and act as though the physical body is all in all, as though it is the only thing worth caring for and thinking about. They exaggerate the importance of the physical and become its abject slaves.

The physical body is the lowest and least intelligent of the different principles making up the human entity. Yet people allow their minds and their souls to become dominated and terrified by the sensations of the physical body.

When the servants in the house control and terrify the master, when the master becomes their slave and they can do with him as they please, there cannot be order and harmony in that house.

We must expect the same results when the lower principles in Man lord it over the higher. When physical weakness, illness and pain fill the mind with fear and dismay, reason becomes clouded, the will atrophied and self-control is lost.

Every thought and every emotion has its direct effect upon the physical constituents of the body. The mental and emotional vibrations become physical vibrations and structures. Discord in the mind is translated into physical disease in the body, while the harmonies of hope, faith, cheerfulness, happiness, love and altruism create in the organism the corresponding health vibrations.

Have you ever noticed how the written or printed notes of a tone piece or the perforations on the paper music roll of an automatic player are arranged in symmetrical and geometrical figures and groups? Dry sand strewn on the top of a piano on which harmonious tone combinations are produced shows a tendency to arrange itself in symmetrical patterns.

In this you have a visual illustration of the translation of harmonious sound vibrations, which express the harmonics of the soul's emotions, into correspondingly harmonious arrangements and configurations in the physical material of the paper roll.

A jumble of discords of sound, if reproduced on a music roll, would present a chaotic jumble of perforations.

Thus the purely mental and emotional is translated into its corresponding discords or harmonies in the physical.

As the perforations on the paper music roll arrange themselves either symmetrically or without symmetry and order, in strict accordance with the harmonies or discords of the composition, so the atoms, molecules and cells in the physical body group themselves in normal or abnormal structures of health or of disease in exact correspondence with the harmonious or the discordant vibrations conveyed to them from the mental and emotional planes.

Another Illustration: Two violins, as they leave the shop of the maker, are exactly alike in material, structure and quality of tone. One of the two instruments is constantly used by beginners and persons incapable of producing pure notes. The other passes into the hands of an artist who understands how to use the instrument to the best advantage and who draws from it only musical tones that are true in pitch and quality.

After a few years, compare the two violins again. You will find that the one used by the tyros in music has deteriorated in its musical qualities, while the one in the hands of the artist has greatly improved in quality and purity of tone. What is the reason? The atoms and molecules in the wood of the two instruments have grouped themselves according to the discords or the harmonies that have been produced from them.

If this rearrangement of atoms is possible in dead wood, how much easier must be this adjustment of atoms, molecules and cells to discordant or harmonious vibratory influence in the living, plastic and fluidic human organism!

What harmony is to music, hope, faith, cheerfulness, happiness, sympathy, love and altruism are to the vibratory conditions of the human entity. These emotions are in alignment with the constructive principle in Nature. They harmonize the physical vibrations, relax the tissues and open them wide to the inflow of the life force.

Swedenborg truly says: "The warmth of life is the heat of the divine love permeating and animating the universe." The more we possess of hope, faith, love and their kindred emotions, the more we open our-selves to the inflow and action of the vital energies. The good-natured, cheerful, sympathetic person is more alive than the crabbed, morose or selfish individual.

It has been proved over and over again by everyday experience that **mental and emotional conditions positively affect the chemical composition of the tissues and secretions of the body.** The destructive emotions of fear, worry, anger, jealousy, revengeful-ness, envy, etc., actually poison the fluids and tissues of the body. The bite of an angry man may cause blood-poisoning and prove as fatal as the bite of a mad dog. Sudden fear, anger or any other destructive emo-tion in the nursing mother may cause illness or even death of the infant.

In psychological laboratories it has been found by scientifically conducted experiments that under the influence of destructive mental and emotional conditions, the secretions and excretions of the body show an increase of morbid and poisonous elements.

Selfishness, fear and worry contract and congeal the blood vessels, the nerve fibers, and the other channels through which the life forces are conveyed from the innermost source of life to different parts and or-gans of the physical body. The flow of the life currents is impeded and diminished. Such are the actual physiological effects of fear, anxiety and egotism on the physical organism.

A man under the influence of great fear and one exposed to freez-ing present the same outward appearance. In both cases death may re-sult through the congealing of the tissues and the shutting out of the life currents. The person afflicted with the worry habit may not die sud-denly like the one overcome by great and sudden fear. Nevertheless, the fear and worry vibrations maintained constantly will surely obstruct and diminish the inflow of the life force, lower the vitality and there-with the resistance to the encroachment of influences inimical to the health of the organism.

The cells in the body are negative, or, at least, they should be negative to the positive mind. The relationship of the mind to the cell should be like that of hypnotist to subject. If the mind could not ex-ert such absolute control over the cells and cell groups, it would be im-possible for us to walk, talk, write, dodge danger, etc., with almost automatic ease.

The cells are not able to reason upon the truth or untruth of the suggestions conveyed to them from the mind. They accept its promptings unqualifiedly and act accordingly.

Thus, if the mind constantly thinks of, say, the stomach as being in a badly diseased condition, unable to do its work properly, the mental images of weakness and disease with their accompanying fear vibrations are telegraphed over the efferent nerves to the cells of the stomach and these become more and more weakened and diseased through the destructive vibrations sent to them from the mind.

I often advise my patients to procure a book on anatomy and physiology and to study and keep constantly before their mind's eye the normal structure and functions of a healthy stomach or liver or whatever organ may be involved in any particular case.

Positive Affirmations

This explains why affirmations of health are justified in the face of disease. The health conditions must be first established in the mind before they can be conveyed to and impressed upon the cells.

The well-being of the human body as a whole depends upon the health of the billions of minute cells which compose it. These cells are so small that they have to be magnified several hundred times under a powerful microscope before we can see them. Yet they are independent living beings which grow, assimilate food, multiply and die like the big cell, Man.

These little cells are congregated in communities which form the organs and tissues of the body and in these communities they carry on the complicated activities of citizens living in a large city. Some are carriers, bringing food materials to the tissues and organs or conveying waste and morbid matter to the excretory channels of the body. Other cells manufacture chemical substances, such as sugar, fats, ferments, hormones etc., for the production of which man requires complicated factories. Still others act as policemen and soldiers which protect the commonwealth against bacteria, parasites and other hostile invaders.

The marvelous work performed by these little organisms, as well as observations made in the dissecting room and under the microscope, strongly indicate that these cells are endowed with some sort of individual intelligence. They do their work without our aid or conscious volition. But, nevertheless, they are greatly influenced by the varying conditions of the mind. While their activities seem to be controlled through the sympathetic nervous system, they stand in direct telegraphic communication with headquarters in the brain and every impulse of the mind is conveyed to them.

If there be dismay and confusion in the mind, this condition is telegraphically conveyed over the nerve trunks and filaments to every cell in the body, and as a result these little workers and soldiers become panic-stricken and incapable of rightly performing their manifold duties.

The cell system of the body resembles a vast army. The mind is the general at the head of it. The cells are the soldiers, divided into groups for special work.

Much of the work of an army is carried on through different well-established departments, as the commissariat, the hospital service, the scouts and pickets, etc. Though the life and the activities of the army are so well regulated that they seem automatic, nevertheless much depends upon the commander.

The vital processes of the human organism, digestion, assimilation, elimination, respiration, the circulation of the blood, etc., are going on without our volition, whether we be awake or asleep. These involuntary activities are impelled by the **sympathetic** nervous system, while the voluntary functions of the body are controlled through the **motor** [voluntary] nervous system. This division, however, is not a sharp one, and the two departments frequently overlap one another.

The sympathetic nervous system resembles the commissarial department of the army, which attends to the material welfare of the soldiers, while the motor nervous system, with headquarters in the brain, corresponds to the commander with his executive staff, the nerve centers in the spinal cord and other parts of the body being the subordinate officers in the field.

While the physical well-being of the army depends upon the almost automatic work of its different departments, its mind and soul is the man commanding it. He determines the spirit, the energy and the efficiency of the vast organization.

If the commander-in-chief lacks insight, force and determination, the discipline of the army will be lax and its efficiency greatly impaired. If he is a craven, without faith in himself and in the cause he represents, his lack of courage, his doubt and indecision will communicate themselves to the whole army, resulting in discouragement and defeat.

The most successful commanders have been those who were possessed of absolute confidence in themselves and in the efficiency of their army, who in the face of gravest danger and discouraging situations pressed on to the predetermined goal with dogged courage and resolution. Determination and pertinacity of this kind create the magnetic power which imparts itself to every individual soldier in the army and makes him a willing subject, even unto death, to the will of his commander.

When the plague was invading Napoleon's army, that great general entered the hospitals where the victims of the plague were lying, took them by the hand and conversed with them. He did this to overcome the fear in the hearts of his soldiers, and thus to protect them against the dread disease. He said: "A man whose will can conquer the world, can conquer the plague."

To my mind, this was one of the greatest deeds of the Corsican. At a time when "New Thought" was practically unknown, the genius of this man had grasped its principles and was making them factors in his apparent success. "Apparent" because, while we admire his genius, we deplore the ends to which he applied his wonderful powers.

At times when the battle seemed lost, Napoleon would go to the front where the danger was greatest; and by the mere sight of him the hard-pressed soldiers under his command were inspired to super-human effort and final victory.

As long as the glamour of invincibility surrounded him, Napoleon **was invincible,** because he infused into his soldiers a faith and courage which nothing could withstand. But when the cunning of the Russian broke his power and decimated his ranks on the ice-bound steppes, the hypnotic spell was broken also. Friends and enemies alike recognized that, after all, he was but a man, subject to chance and circumstance; and from that time on he was vulnerable and suffered defeat after defeat.

The power of the mind over the physical body and its involuntary functions (the functions which are regulated and controlled through the sympathetic nervous system) may be illustrated by the demonstrated facts of hypnotism. Through the exertion of his own imagination and his will-power, the hypnotist can so dominate the brain and through the brain the physical body of his subject, as to influence not only the sensory functions, but also heart action and respiration. By the power of his will the hypnotist is able to retard or accelerate pulse and respiration, and even to subdue the heart beat so that it becomes hardly perceptible.

If it is possible thus to control by the power of will the vital functions in the body of another person, it must be possible also to control these functions in our own bodies. Many a Hindu fakir and yogi have developed this power of the mind over the physical body to a marvelous extent.

Here lies the true domain of mental therapeutics. We can learn to dominate and regulate the vital activities and the life currents in our bodies so that they will do their work intelligently and serenely even under the stress of illness or of danger. We can, by the power of will, direct the vital currents to those parts and organs which need them most and we can relieve congested areas by equalizing the circulation, by drawing from the surplus of blood and nerve currents and distributing the vital fluids over other parts of the body.

We must be careful, however, to use our higher powers in conformity with Nature's intent; that is, we must not endeavor to suppress Nature's cleansing and healing efforts. It is possible to do this by the power of will as well as with ice bags and drugs.

Mentally and emotionally, as well as physically, we must work **with** Nature, not against her. When we understand the fundamental laws of disease and cure, we cannot well do otherwise.

CHAPTER XXXIX

HOW SHALL WE PRAY?

Shall we say: "Father, give me this Father, do for me that!"? Or shall we say: "Behold, I am perfect! Imperfection, sin and suffering are only errors of mortal mind!"?

Or shall we pray: "Father, give me of Thy strength that I may live in harmony with Thy law, for thus only will all good come to me!"?

The first way is to beg, the second, to steal, the third, to earn by honest effort.

"Father, give me this "—**"Father do for me that "** Thus prayed our fathers, not understanding the great law of compensation, the law of giving and receiving, which demands that we give an equivalent for everything we receive. To receive without giving is to beg.

The lily, in return for the nourishment it receives from the soil and the sun, gives its beauty and fragrance. The birds of the air give a return for their sustenance by their songs, their beauty of plumage, and by destroying worms and insects, the enemies of plants and men. Every living thing gives an equivalent for its existence in some way or other.

With Man, the fulfillment of the law of service and of compensation becomes conscious and voluntary, and his self-respect refuses to take without giving.

"Behold, I am perfect Imperfection, sin, and suffering are only errors of mortal mind " Such is the prayer of certain metaphysical healers.

To assume the possession of goodness and perfection without an earnest effort to develop and to deserve these qualities, means to steal the glory of the only Perfect One. The assumption of present perfection precludes the necessity of striving and laboring for its attainment. If I am already all goodness, all love, all wisdom, and all power, what remains for me to strive for?

Herein lies the danger of metaphysical idealism. While it may dispel pessimism, fear, and anxiety, it inevitably weakens the will power and the capacity for self-help and personal effort.

The ideal of the metaphysician is the ideal of the animal. The animal does not worry about right or wrong, nor, with few exceptions, does it make provision for the future. Its care and forethought extend only to the next meal. But this perfect, ideal, passive trust in Nature's bounty causes the animal to remain animal and prevents its rising above the narrow limitations of habit and instinct.

The inherent faculties, capacities, and powers of the human soul can be developed only by effort and use. The savage, living in the most favored regions of the earth, depending for his sustenance in perfect faith and trust on Nature's never-failing bounty, has remained savage. Through ages he has risen but little above the level of the beasts that perish.

The great law of use ordains that those faculties and powers which we do not develop remain in abeyance, and that those which we possess weaken and atrophy if we fail to exercise them.

The Master, Jesus, emphasized this law of use in many of his parables and sayings.

"For whosoever hath, to him shall be given, and he shall have more abundance: but whosoever hath not, from him shall be taken away even that he hath."

What does this mean? Those who have the desire and the will to work out their own salvation, acquire greater knowledge and power in exact proportion to their well-directed efforts; but those who have neither the desire nor the will to help themselves, lose their natural endowments and the possibilities and opportunities which these would have conferred upon them.

The anatomy and physiology of the human brain reveal the fact that for every voluntary faculty, capacity, and power of body, mind, and soul which we wish to develop, we have to create new cells and centers in the brain. In this respect, Nature gives us no more and no less than we deserve and work for. If we "try to cheat" by usurping the perfection and the power which we have not honestly earned and developed, then sometime, somewhere we shall have to "square the balance. "

The Right Way to Pray

After all, the only true prayer is personal effort and self-help. This does not mean that we should not invoke the help of the Higher Powers, of those who have gone before us, of the Great Friends and Invisible Helpers, and of the Great Father, the giver of all life, all wisdom, and all power. But **we should pray for strength to do our work, not to have it done for us.** The wise parent will not do for the child the home tasks assigned him at school. Neither will the powers on high or the Great Friends perform our allotted tasks for us.

This life is a school for personal effort. If it were not so, life would be meaningless. From the cradle to

the grave,, our days are one continuous effort to learn, to acquire, to overcome difficulties. Only in this way can we develop our latent faculties, capacities, and powers. These cannot be developed by having our tasks done for us, nor by assuming that we already know and possess everything.

The athlete must do his own training. No one else can do it for him. The **assumption** of superiority over his opponent will riot develop his suppleness of body and strength of muscle. To be sure, faith and courage are essential to victory, but they must be backed by careful and persistent training. Vainglorious boasting alone will not win the contest.

So in the battle of life, the more faith we have in God, in the Great Friends, and in our own powers, the wider do we open ourselves to the inflow of wisdom and strength from all that is good and true and powerful in the universe. But through persistent and welldirected effort alone can we control the powers and fashion the materials which Nature has so lavishly bestowed upon us.

The creative will, actuated by desire and enlightened by reason, brings order and harmony out of chaotic forces and materials. And yet certain metaphysicians tell us that we ourselves must do nothing to overcome weakness, sin, and suffering, that we must depend entirely upon the efficiency of metaphysical formulas, that the deity and the powers of Nature are jealous of our personal efforts, that we must not try to help ourselves lest we forfeit their good will.

Is it not blasphemous to assume that God would blame us and withhold his aid because we dared to use the faculties, capacities, and powers with which he has endowed us? You say, "Nobody is foolish enough to claim such things." But this is the teaching of a powerful healing-cult. Its members are forbidden, on penalty of expulsion, to use in the treatment of human ailments the most innocent natural remedies. The giving of an enema, or the common-sense regulation of diet are regarded as sufficient to nullify the power of their metaphysical formulas and to prevent the working of Nature's healing forces.

One of our patients who had been under such treatment until she was in a dying condition, told us afterwards that her bowels often did not move for a week, and that, when she complained to her "healer" about this condition and asked permission to take an enema, he answered her: "Pay no attention. The Lord is taking care of that in some other way."

The man who said this had been a prominent allopathic physician before he turned "healer." He, too, like so many others ignorant of Nature's simple laws, had swung from one extreme to the other, from allopathic overdoing to metaphysical underdoing. In this instance, the Lord "took care" of the patient's bowels until she was taken down with a severe attack of appendicitis and peritonitis.

Amidst all the extremes, Nature Cure points the common-sense middle way. Basing its teachings and its practices on a clear understanding of the laws of health, disease, and cure, it refrains from suppressing acute diseases with poisonous drugs or the knife, realizing that they are in reality Nature's cleansing and healing efforts. Neither does it sit idly by and expect the Lord, or metaphysical formulas, or the medicine bottle and the knife, to do our work and to make good for our violations of Nature's laws.

Understanding the Law, Nature Cure believes in cooperating with the law; in giving the Lord a helping hand. It teaches that "God helps him who helps himself," that He will not become angry and refuse His help if His children use rightly the reason, the willpower, and the self-control with which he has endowed them, so that they may achieve their own salvation.

Nature Cure from beginning to end is one grand, true prayer. It teaches The Law on all planes of being, the physical, the mental, the moral, and the spiritual; and it insists that the only way to attain perfect health of body, mind, and soul is to comply with the law to the best of our ability. **When we do that, we place ourselves in alignment with the constructive principle in Nature, and in exact proportion to our intelligent and voluntary co-operation with the laws of our being, all good things will come to us.**

Therefore we pray: "Father, give me of Thy strength that I may live in harmony with Thy law, for thus only will all good come to me."

Chapter XL

Scientific Relaxation and Normal Suggestion

Under the strain of work-a-day hurry and worry, your nerve vibrations are apt to become more and more intense and excited. They run away with you until, as the saying goes, "you are flying all to pieces."

A good illustration of this condition of the nervous system may be found in a team of horses shying at some object in their path. The driver, panic-stricken, has dropped the reins, the frightened horses have taken the bits between their teeth and are dashing headlong down the road, until their master regains control, checks the animals in their maddened course, and compels them to resume their ordinary pace.

So the high-strung, oversensitive individual must gain control over his nervous system and must subdue his runaway mental and emotional activities into restful, harmonious vibrations.

This is done by **insuring sufficient rest** and **sleep** under the right conditions and by **practicing scientific relaxation** at all times.

The "nervous" person gets easily excited. Comparatively little things will cause an outbreak of intense irritation or emotional hyperactivity.

Usually, the victim of unbalanced nerves is of the high-strung, sensitive type, naturally inclining to more rapid vibrations on all planes, capable of greater achievement than the stolid, heavy, slow-vibrating person who doesn't know that he has any nerves, but he is also in greater danger of mental and emotional overstrain and physical depletion as a result of the excessive and uncontrolled expenditure of life force and nervous energy.

Relaxation while Working

At first glance this expression may seem paradoxical, but experience will teach that it is not only possible, but absolutely necessary that we perform our work in a relaxed and serene condition of body and mind. The most strenuous physical or mental labor will then not cause as much exhaustion as light work done in a state of nervous tension, irritability, fretfulness or worry.

Relaxation while working necessitates planning and sys-

tem. Most nervous breakdowns result not so much from overwork as from the vitality wasted through lack of orderly procedure. Therefore, take some time to plan and arrange your work and form the habit of doing certain things that have to be done every day as nearly as possible in the same way (making sure that it is the right way) and at the same time of the day. Such orderly system will soon become habitual and result in saving much valuable time and energy.

Always cultivate a serene and cheerful attitude of mind and soul, taking whatever comes as part of the day's work, doing your best under the circumstances, but absolutely refusing to worry and fret about anything. Do not cross a bridge before you get to it, and do not waste time regretting something that cannot be undone.

Relaxation while Sitting

Sit upright in a comfortable chair without strain or tension, spine and head erect, the legs forming right angles with the thighs (the chair should be neither too high nor too low), feet resting firmly upon the floor, toes pointing slightly outward, the forearms resting lightly upon the legs with the hands upon the knees. This must be accomplished without effort, for effort means tension.

Dismiss all thoughts of hurry, care, worry or fear and dwell upon the following thoughts:

"I am now completely relaxed in body and mind. I am receptive to Nature's harmonious and invigorating vibrations—they dispel the discordant and destructive vibrations of hurry, worry, fear and anger. New life, new health, new strength are entering into me with every breath, pervading my whole being."

Repeat these thoughts mentally, or, if it helps you, say them aloud several times, quietly and forcefully, impressing them deeply upon your inner consciousness.

After practicing relaxation in this manner, lie down for a few minutes' rest—if circumstances permit—or practice rhythmical breathing (see Chapter Twenty-Eight). Then return to your work and endeavor to maintain a calm, trustful, controlled attitude of mind.

If you are inclined to be irritable, suspicious, jealous, fault-finding, envious, etc., dwell on the following thought pictures:

"I am now fully relaxed, at rest and at peace. The world is an echo. If I send forth irritable, suspicious, hateful thought vibrations, the like will return to me from other minds. I shall

think such thoughts no longer. God is love, love is harmony, happiness, heaven. The more I send forth Love, the more I am like God; the more of love will God and men return to me; the more shall I realize true happiness, true health, true strength and true success."

Relaxation Before Going to Sleep

When ready to go to sleep, lie flat on your back, so that as nearly as possible every part of the spine touches the bed, extend the arms along the sides of the body, hands turned upward, palms open, every muscle relaxed. Dismiss all thoughts of work, annoyance or anxiety. Say to yourself: "I am now going to sleep soundly and peacefully. I am master of my body, my mind and my soul. Nothing evil shall disturb me. At ___ A. M., neither earlier nor later, I shall awaken rested and refreshed, strong in body and mind. I shall meet tomorrow's tasks and duties promptly and serenely."

Simple as this formula may seem, it has helped cure many a case of persistent insomnia and nervous prostration. Having thus set your mental alarm clock, with a few times, practice you will be able to wake up, without being called, at the appointed time and to demonstrate to yourself the power of your mind over your body.

The quality of your sleep and its effect upon your system depend on the character of the mental and psychic vibrations carried into it. If you harbor thoughts of passion, worry or fear, these destructive thought vibrations will disturb your slumbers and you will awaken in the morning weak and tired. If, however, you repeat mentally a formula such as the above, suggesting harmonious, constructive thoughts, until you lose consciousness, you will carry into your slumbers vibrations of rest, health and strength, producing corresponding effects upon the physical organism.

After a perfectly relaxed condition of body and mind has been attained, it is not necessary to remain lying on the back. Any position of the body may then be assumed which seems most restful.

My patients frequently ask what position of the body is best during sleep. It is not good to lie continuously in any one position. This tends to cause unsymmetrical development of the different parts of the body and to affect unfavorably the functions of various organs. It is best to change occasionally from one position to another, as bodily comfort seems to indicate and require.

Many persons fret and worry if sleep does not come as quickly as desired. They picture to themselves in darkest colors the dire results of wakefulness. Such a state of mind makes sleep impossible. If persisted in, it will inevitably lead to chronic insomnia.

Instead of indulging in hurtful worry, say to yourself: "I do not care whether I sleep or not! Though I do not sleep, I am lying here perfectly relaxed, at rest and at peace. I am strengthened and rested by remaining in a state of peaceful relaxation."

However, the "I do not care" must be actually meant and felt, must not be merely a mechanical repetition of words.

Nothing is more conducive to sleep, even under the most trying circumstances, than such an "I-don't-care" attitude of mind. Try it, and the chances are that just because you do not care, you will fall fast asleep.

Chapter XLI

Conclusion

Our critics say: "If Nature Cure is all that you claim for it, why is it not more generally accepted by the medical profession and the public?"

The greatest drawback to spreading the Nature Cure idea is **the necessity of self-control which it imposes.** If our cures of so-called incurable diseases could be made without asking the patients to change their habits of living, without the demand of effort on their own part, Nature Cure sanitariums could not be built fast enough in this country.

No matter how marvelous the results of the natural methods—when investigators learn that the treatment necessitates the control of indiscriminate appetite and self-indulgence and the persistent practice of natural living and all that this involves, they exclaim: "The natural regimen may be all right, but who can live up to it? You are asking the impossible. You are looking for a perfection which does not exist. Your directions call for an amount of willpower and self-control which nobody possesses."

Fortunately, however, this is not true. Human nature is good enough and strong enough to comply with Nature's laws. Furthermore, the natural ways must be the most pleasant in the end or Nature is a fraud and a cheat. True enjoyment of life and happiness are impossible without perfect physical, mental and moral health and these depend upon natural living and **natural** treatment of human ailments.

Strengthening of Will-Power and Self-Control

If I were asked the question: "What do you consider the greatest benefit to be derived from the Nature Cure regimen?" I should answer: **"The strengthening of willpower and self-control."**

This is the very purpose of life. Upon it depends all further achievement. Self-control is the master's key to all higher development on the mental, moral and spiritual planes of being; but before we can exercise it on the higher planes, we must have learned to apply it on the lower plane, in the management and control of our physical appetites and habits. When we have learned to control these, higher development will come easy.

A good method for strengthening the willpower is autosuggestion. The most opportune moments in the twenty-four hours of the day for practicing this mental magic are those before dropping to sleep. At this time there is the least disturbance and interference from outside influences, the mind is most passive and susceptible to suggestion and impressions made under these favorable conditions upon the "phonograph records" of the subconscious mind are the most lasting and the most powerful to control physical, mental and moral activities.

When thoroughly relaxed, at rest and at peace, say to yourself: "Whatever duties confront me tomorrow, I shall execute them promptly, without wavering or hesitation. I shall not give in to this bad habit which has been controlling me. I shall do that only of which reason and conscience approve."

In order to be more specific and systematic and to obtain results more surely and quickly, **concentrate upon one weakness at a time.** When that has been overcome, take up another one, until in this way you have attained perfect control over your thoughts, feelings and actions.

Suppose you have acquired the habit of remaining in bed and dozing after your mental alarm clock has given its signal to arise and you dread the effort of going through your morning exercises and ablutions. Then, the night before, impress upon the subconscious mind deeply and firmly the following suggestions: "Tomorrow morning, on awakening, I shall jump out of bed without hesitation and go through my morning exercises with zest and vigor."

Or, suppose you are subject to the fear and worry habit. Say to yourself: "Tomorrow or any time thereafter when depressing, gloomy thoughts threaten to control me, I shall overcome them with thoughts of hope and faith, and with absolute confidence in the Divine power of the will within me to overcome and to achieve."

In this manner you may give the subconscious mind suggestions and impressions for overcoming bad habits and for establishing and strengthening good habits.

If a serious problem is confronting you, and you are unable to solve it to your satisfaction, think upon it just before you are dropping off to sleep and confidently demand that the right solution come to you during the hours of rest. The inner consciousness is always awake. It is the watchman who awakens you at the appointed time in the morning. It will work upon your problem while your physical brain is asleep. In this lies the psychological justification for the popular phrase: "Before I decide the matter I'll sleep over it."

In the practice of mental magic, as in everything else, success depends upon patience and perseverance. It would be entirely useless to go through these mental drills occasionally and in a desultory fashion; but if persisted in faithfully and intelligently, they will prove truly magical in their effects upon the development of willpower and self-control, and on these depend the mastery of conditions within and without, the conquest of fate and destiny.

LaVergne, TN USA
08 September 2010
196347LV00005B/102/A